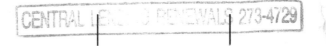
Fit, Healthy
&
Intoxicated

Fit, Healthy
&
Intoxicated

A self-help book for alcohol lovers

by Cindy Cannon

Published by Brolga Publishing Pty Ltd
ABN 46 063 962 443
PO Box 12544
A'Beckett Street
Melbourne VIC 8006
e-mail: bepublished@brolgapublishing.com.au

National Library of Australia CIP

Cannon, Cindy.
Fit, healthy and intoxicated: a self-help book for alcohol lovers
ISBN 1 920785 33 7
1. Drinking of alcoholic beverages — Health aspects. c. Alcohol - Health aspects. I. Title.

Printed in China
Cover design by Trish Hart
Typeset by Diana Evans

contents

foreword

Having been asked to do the foreword for this book creates a conflict in interest — to praise a story about one of my patients who has always oozed vitality and a positive approach to her health and life, and to link this to the use of alcohol which more often than not is one of our medical demons.

When I first met Cindy over 8 years ago she always walked in with a smile, an interesting anecdote and by the way a nuisance thing called a medical problem which she wanted to eradicate immediately!! Or at least as soon as possible.

She was always in a hurry, as if life is far too important, and can be lots of fun, to let minor health things get in the way, so her visits were not very frequent. Despite these infrequent visits I was able to quickly learn she had a quirky nature with a strong drive for moving on with her life.

This came to a climax when she presented one day and openly stated her apparent overuse of alcohol, but decided she had better have some tests to see how much damage it was doing to her. With her description of her daily use I was fairly pessimistic about the outcome of the results, knowing that a female's tolerance to alcohol is far less than that of a male. After the blood was taken I waited to see how bad the news would be, and how she would need to quell her exuberance and make fairly dramatic changes to her daily routine. I was stunned to say the least when the results came back, and as I sat there going through them with her I could see the glow in her eyes sparkle and the width of her smile grow.

I am ethically and morally bound to warn people of the dangers of alcohol, especially in excess use, the damage it does to our body and the association with depression, disinhibition, violence and the disastrous effects when it tries to drive a motor car. I will not sway from this.

The reason I agreed to comment on this book, is that Cindy displays something that I have spent years fine tuning in my counselling and health management skills, trying to impart a tiny part of the importance of quality of a person's life; how to deal with adversity, overcome fear and grief, and move on with one's life to attain a sense of satisfaction, peacefulness and fulfilment. I believe Cindy exemplifies this as she has positivity, mixed in with a cheeky sense of humour and her routine incorporates the enjoyment of alcohol. As I said this is a precarious mix and defies usual medical advice, but the sense of her vitality and the wellness she exudes is the reason that I am so impressed by her story. She wants to live life to the fullest, create enjoyment and happiness within that life, and not shirk her responsibilities that she knows are there. This is the essence of life that I have tried for years to instil into sad and unhappy people, who struggle to find a glimmer of hope in their life. Perhaps reading this book would give them a chance to rethink their own life, and create another happy person.

Dr Graeme Baro

M.B.,B.S. (Monash)

Fit, Healthy and Intoxicated

1
graduation

I'm so pleased with myself. I recently spent nearly two months in the heart of the magnificent red desert in north-west South Australia, working with my partner Mark and father Deane on an interesting Aboriginal land rights case. It was a big deal, with an entourage of lawyers, barristers, court staff. As the court reporters, we could party with almost anyone — and did!

Mark and I did our most serious drinking with the Marla Travellers Rest staff, particularly the young ones who cleaned the rooms, worked in the kitchen etc. But in a generous display of evenhandedness, we also drank and socialised with the great array of people associated with the court, from drivers to IT people, interpreters to QCs and professors of anthropology. We made many wonderful and interesting friends.

This is a self-help book for all you excellent people out there who also love to drink habitually and party with friends (or on your own), celebrate life and enjoy it to the max, making the most of every day, but still get up early enough to go to work, preferably without a hangover. I have hundreds of friends and relatives in need of this book. Fortunately I'm an expert in the field and have lots of good news about effective ways to maximise drinking pleasure and minimise damage.

Now returning to my example above and why I started with Marla. The thing I haven't yet mentioned is that most of us involved with the hearing nearly worked ourselves to death. We rarely had a day off and often worked till around midnight, with many early starts.

Our bodies and minds were exhausted most of the time due to late work finishes and even later bedtimes. My eyes were half-blinded by laptop screens, fine red dust and lack of sleep. All this brain-draining work and stress, plus making all these great new friends and just wanting to drink, talk and party with them — every day was like two-in-one. And no matter how tired, stressed etc I was, even in the tough times I was happy. So I worked like a dog, partied daily and survived well. At about 40 and leaving 20 years of heavy drinking in my wake, I reckon that qualifies me as an expert!

II
the A word

Alcoholic. Enough to scare many people into facial contortions normally reserved for utter contempt. But it's just another A word, like Attitude. It's your attitude, not the word, that packs the punch. I suspect the tendency for Aussies to recoil with shock, horror, indignation and heavy judgmentalism at the mere concept of alcoholism has its roots in history and our enthusiastic embracing of all things American. Think Abolition.

I'm over it. Sure, I can understand why so many people react with alarm when I call myself an alcoholic. They can cope with the word "alcohol" without a stress response, but add the "ic" and they're running for cover. You'd think it was contagious. From my perspective, this is quite amusing, tempting me to yell from the rooftops, "I'm an alcoholic!" But I can resist a temptation that might attract men in uniform.

What people are running from is fear: fear that they may be an ic themselves or may become one if exposed to dangerous radicals like myself; fear that to be an ic is to be useless, disgraceful, prone to embarrassing honesty and lack of social airs, possibly smelly, braindead

7

and likely to vomit, a drain on society; fear that drinking more than X drinks per day/week will lead to holus-bolus shedding of moral standards and such disinterest in one's own life that inevitably job, family and all else will be lost in an orgy of gambling or other frown-worthy pursuits.

The sad thing about such stereotyping is there are victims. People who barely drink enough to exercise the liver are suffering unnecessary guilt trips, and those who should be treating well-worn livers with respect are not even prepared to admit it. On top of this, the self-right-eous are given a green light to carry on tormenting oth-ers. But do you need someone else to tell you what or who you are? Do you normally let others dictate what's right for you? Don't you have a right to be ic?

I'm exercising my ic rights to the full, and heaven help the do-gooder who tries to stop me. (Ever seen an alco in danger of losing their drink?) If the need-a-life brigade must expend their energy criticising others, so be it. They won't change my attitude. I can do without the self-flagellation. Such an extraordinary amount of human effort is devoted to guilt-tripping. It seems like madness, but it's just conditioning. Our parents did it, their parents did it etc. It's not easy and you may need to fight like a warrior, but it is possible to break the habit. It takes knowledge (identify the problem) and time to change (practise). In warrior-speak, identify enemy, then fight with Death Before Dishonour vigour. See chapter XVIII for a few pointers.

All this said, however, you may find it unbearable to describe yourself as an alcoholic. If so, don't. Call yourself a heavy drinker, a social drinker, even a teetotaller if it makes you feel good. What you DO is more telling than what you say. Words don't change anything. The important thing is not to give yourself a hard time, no matter what your preferred self-description may be.

After all, what is an ic? Who is to say one definition is the correct one? Am I an alcoholic because I love to drink, because I don't like to stop once I've started, because I drink every day, because it's part of my routine, my lifestyle, because I'm psychologically dependent? How can I even know that I am an alcoholic? Answer: who cares. These are just words.

When I devised this book in my mind it was called The Healthy Alcoholic. The title fits, because it is about how to be just that. In uncharacteristically sheepish fashion, however, I changed the name to cater for those who fear the ic. It would be a shame to scare readers off before they opened the cover, as a good friend pointed out. I'm hoping by the end, however, you'll have a revised attitude and will feel more ic-friendly (even more warrior-like).

Fear of association with the A word is doubtless the reason a barrister friend (who saves his warrior for court) declined my invitation to write an "about the author" (make that "alcoholic") foreword. He seemed ideal, having seen me in action, working (to excess) and drinking (ditto), and could vouch for my expertise in both fields. Being a QC, I thought this would look great at the start of my book, giving it a weighty credibility. But imagine if putting his name on an A-word book shattered his career and he sued me in court! I'd be a goner.

Things are looking pretty bleak already. I'm bound to offend numerous people, groups, corporations and industries (might hide book from them), not to mention relatives. It's not that I want to, but it's inevitable. My views on alcoholism are not politically correct. They're not even medically sound. But all the doctors in the world won't convince me it's not possible to be a healthy alcoholic. I've been one for decades, and it's my privilege to know many others with even greater experience.

Something important has to be said here and it may give me a leg to stand on if I'm sued in court for publishing misleading information. (That warrior-like QC could be a judge by now.) This book is based on personal experience. I'm not a doctor. The only degree I have is a BA and it was in the social sciences. I'm just a court reporter with a wealth of drinking experience, in very good health and enjoying a lifestyle that suits me perfectly. My knowledge of food, the body and exercise is based upon reading, experience and experimentation.

While I like to think of myself as an amateur psychologist, having witnessed and experienced mind malfunctions and having undergone various stress therapies that actually work, again I have no formal training. This won't stop me making suggestions about ways to make your mind a more positive place.

Like most people, I've had bad times in my life. Probably the worst was during my early thirties, when I started getting really hot and red at work. It happened every day. Each morning I'd wake up and reassure myself, "Don't worry, you feel okay now, you'll be right today," but then I'd arrive at the office and it was as if the airconditioning triggered an exaggerated heat response, turning me into a beetroot. I was embarrassed and worried, not understanding what was going on. Although it only happened at work, I resisted the temptation to leave and try another job. Somehow I knew the problem originated within.

For two and a half years the red face symptom continued. I could hardly drink beer quickly enough when I got home, and usually felt happy for the first time all day once I'd downed half a dozen. After at least a year of desperately wishing it away (and failing), I started seeing doctors and a naturopath. Eventually a diagnosis was plain: stress. Other than crying, I had no idea how to deal with this or why it had happened.

It took years to really get better. I had herbal

remedies and acupuncture, took up yoga, saw a beautiful alternative therapist woman who gave me cool-down feel-good meditation exercises and taught me about the players in my mind. She explained that it had taken up to 30 years to get into such a state of stress, so it wasn't going to be cured in a day. Frightfully annoying as this was, of course it was true.

Slowly, with the help of the naturopath and therapist and reading books about stress, the mind etc, I recovered. Even black clouds have a silver lining and suffering makes an awesome teacher, so this was truly a learning experience and in hindsight I'm lucky to have had it. It's easier for me to be happy now, and I understand the nature of stress and our individual reactions to it, plus I possess tools that help me keep my mind positive and be my own best friend.

Think about how plants and seeds love to grow in manure and thrive on it. If suffering is shit, we grow on it too.

My motivation to write this book is born of a genuine belief that I've learnt many practical lessons about drinking and health which will be helpful to others. It would be great to make some money as well, but Mark keeps telling me that endless books are written and almost none are published and blah negative blah. So if it gets published; bonus. If other drinkers learn about being healthier and happier; jackpot.

III
love at first sip

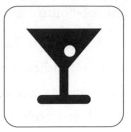

I love drinking. The trick is to find practical ways of staying healthy and avoiding hangovers. Unfortunately, people like me (committed drinkers) are rarely born with this special talent. (Doesn't matter, we have endless others!) When I took to the university tavern with great gusto as soon as the opportunity presented itself, my uni days were filled more with head-throbbing hangovers than lectures.

Back then, at 18 years of age, I didn't realise that fried fatty chips in a sea of salt, enclosed in squishy white bread rolls, were as overwhelming to my then-young liver as the gigantic pints of beer we habitually consumed. At least the beer made me happy. The chip rolls made me feel like I needed a stomach pump.

The only thing I got right in those days was nut munching. I'd encourage you all to eat nuts regularly, particularly good quality ones — brazil nuts, almonds, cashews, walnuts — they're nutrition bombs. Check out your eye whites in the 24 hours following nut consumption — beautifully white, because the body is full of nutrients. Buy nuts fresh, in small quantities to prevent out-of-control gluttony, bloatation and weight gain.

Amongst the stupidest of many idiotic indulgences in those rather messy and embarrassing days was drinking copious amounts of milk as a post-drinking cure, which it wasn't. Little wonder I was covered in pimples and perpetually blowing my nose. Dairy products are made from cow's milk, a super-rich blend of mega-strong nutrients too — but for calves, baby cows, not for humans. Calves grow at a phenomenal rate and cow milk is specially designed for this rapid growth. Your stomach is as different from a cow's, as beer is from Jack Daniels. Your human stomach does not want gluggy cow's milk, and your body does not need it.

Guidelines about dairy products:

• avoid (but don't get religious, it only leads to war)

• cheese is tolerably digestible when eaten with only salad or vegies

• if you have a particular cheese fetish (mine is definitely parmesan) make sure it's good quality and try combining it with stomach artillery (chillis, wine, garlic, dried fruit) to help blast it through the system (the cheese sticks to you because you're irresistible, but that doesn't mean you want to look like cheese)

• white stuff like fetta and ricotta are less risky, especially if eaten with salad or vegies, or in salad sandwiches without butter or mayonnaise (wholemeal or multigrain bread that doesn't defy nature and stay squishy for weeks; you want ingredients from the kitchen, not the science lab)

• cheese with pasta and/or vegies isn't too bad, but you'll probably crash if you have cheese with pasta and meat or fish

• ice cream after a meal will cure insomnia, but good quality home-made styles of ice cream (courtesy of chef, not scientist) are fine on a more or less empty stomach and if not eaten by the container load (as an excess ice cream consumption survivor, I dare not keep any in the fridge. Why haven't the scientific ones developed an ingenious Fridge Safe, to guard against abuse of dangerous substances like this? I suppose the space cadets are too busy playing Star Trek)

• pizzas smothered in cheese are an alarmingly addictive health hazard and will make you fat (or fatter) so if you can't resist pizza pig-outs you'll need a good supply of stomach antacids, most effectively taken an hour or so after the pizza, but in the interim you must work at remaining upright so that gravity is on your side, because after that you'll be snoring (next day's Chronic Fatigue Syndrome is easily explained: all your energy is necessarily committed to digestion, and your liver is working overtime)

I'll try not to bring up dairy products again, in case

the dairy industry decides to sue me. They've got more money than me, which is how they pay for their advertisements. It's interesting that the Japanese traditionally had no dairy products and no word for "menopause" because they didn't get it. They didn't suffer from osteoporosis. Their diet, rich in soy products and seafood, fortified against these conditions.

It's easy to switch to soy milk and even easier to eat tofu, one of my top favourite foods. Even my meat-loving man is into it these days. Buy fresh, rinse in cold water and marinate bite-size finger friendly bits in tamari (similar to soy sauce but yummier and healthier), then enjoy. Your stomach and liver will go wild with delight if you have tofu with mushrooms, broccoli or other vegies, jazzed up with any available herbs, spices, garlic, chilli, ginger. Sausages, meat or seafood can be added if you want a gut-buster.

Alternatively, centimetre-thick slices of tofu under a hot grill will puff up and become chewier, forming a delicious skin; great with well-cooked vegies on top, or layered with other favourite foods in stacks.

Finally, a special warning. There's some extremely dangerous wild parmesan cheese on the market, going under the pseudonym Grana Padana. Scientific classification: Flying Parmie. As the name suggests, it flys. Most commonly occurs whilst cooking, and generally flys straight into mouth, which is always mysteriously open.

Other less lucky FP units spread out and attack the floors and benchtops, like chilling reminders for next morning.

The good news is that the escaped bits decorating the kitchen are clear proof you don't need to go on an emergency diet, although your scales should be discarded immediately if you're silly enough to have any. Focus instead on the abundance of now squished parmie blobs you didn't consume. You've done enough dieting!

I can't even mention the obscenely luscious Reggiano without drooling, or crying because I can't afford it. They make it in Heaven, but fall tragically short of demand. They must have very well paid angels up there, if not lazy ones who spend their lives eating (Reggiano). The only compensation I'm aware of is conjuring up visions of very fat and pimply angels.

IV
beware the turncoats

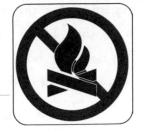

A new chapter, a new tinnie. Almost any time is a good time for a coldie, unless you're already bloated with a gut full of it. If you can't think of any other reason, running out of the previous one will suffice. Right now I'm ready for my third Coopers Sparkling Ale. It's one of my favourites because it's rich and yummy, with a higher-than-usual alcohol content (5.8%) and healthy yeast presence due to being bottle-fermented. Home-brewed beer is extra good also for this reason, although it's hard not to make it a bit too potent. I used to aim for light beer (after a few bouts of rapid onset inebriation). It's a worthwhile and satisfying pursuit to brew your own beer. You need practice and time. It's incredibly cheap.

I'm avoiding my subject because it's slightly painful and unpalatable, and it would feel better to make you all happy with good news. However, it's crucial to be realistic, so I'll fetch my stubbie and dive right in.

Well, shortly. Just had a snack so I don't get too pissed too soon; sourdough bread with honey. I wanted vegemite for the excellent B-vitamins and yeast, but have none. Honey is next best; good sugar pick-me-up. No need for butter or marg — it's easy to get used to. Margarine is not food.

That was yummy so now I'm having more, along with a multi-B vitamin pill because I'll probably drink a lot today, being my non-work Friday and beginning of my weekend. B vitamins are hangover prevention weapons. Think of B as the happy pills, promoting good moods if you're a bit run down. Always take a multi-B vitamin with food if you're in for a big night.

Replenished, I'm ready to continue. At 17 I met Mr X, I think in the uni tavern. That's certainly where our lengthy courtship began. He was older than me, full of general knowledge and political fervour. He taught me about the left side of politics and I became a sort of socialist/Marxist/feminist ball of fury. I thank him for opening my eyes to alternative perspectives and teaching me how to drink way past the dizzy stage. But he was a turncoat.

Like many turncoats, he was frequently the most pop-ular life of the party, very funny, surprising and challenging, often complimentary, a master of manipulation. I was mes-merised. He made me feel lucky and special. Then, through dense rose-coloured glasses, I witnessed a hideous Jekyll and Hyde transformation. His face would almost contort with anger and hatred, which he threw at myself and other friends in venomous words. It was scary.

Mr X couldn't help it. Alcohol gave him an opportunity to vent his anger, and problems not dealt with are landmines. Plus he didn't have the benefit of this book to guide him! So deal with your demons and you won't be a turncoat.

We all need help at times. Counsellors, psychologists and psychiatrists are experts in the mind field, trained to deal with feelings like pain and frustration. If you haven't already suffered and learnt enough to know how to look after and love yourself, try finding someone who's offering solutions which don't take an age, because lying on a couch wallowing in self-pity is fruitless and expensive.

Other medicines for the mind include meditation, yoga, exercise, massage, acupuncture, singing, dancing, tai chi — there are so many great ways to care for yourself. If you have positive thoughts, look on the bright side and don't give yourself a hard time, you can make the most of life.

Some people can't cope with alcohol and/or other drugs. Their heads are too screwy. Self-tormented people can't help torturing others. Aggressive and/or violent people are best avoided. Keep a safe arm's length but polite distance. You can choose the people and situations you embrace in life. Make your own reality — not an original concept. It's probably been outlawed by now, but cigarette papers used to have cute stuff written under the cover. This was my favourite:

"Life is Like Art; You Create Your Own Reality"

The Desiderata wisely suggests:

"Avoid loud and aggressive persons;
   they are vexations to the spirit."

A happy drunk beats a heavy drunk. Fortunately for me, and my drinking buddies, I'm more the loving drunk. When drinking, I love everybody and everything. Sometimes my love extends to bodies in general, and I wonder why on earth I've opted for monogamy. That's one of many good reasons to take Mark to parties; it ensures that Mark is the one who takes me home. Plus he's big and strong, for those rare but dicey occasions when remaining vertical, or functional in any relevant sense, is off the menu.

Thankfully, Mark has rarely been legless, due no doubt to his ample size. Unfortunately, at such times there's no option but to leave him in situ. On one memorable occasion this meant the stairway to the huge town hall where other more mobile revellers were dancing the Zorba at my sister's wedding! Mercifully (as if he didn't have enough to contend with) Mark could only grasp the broad gist of communications bestowed upon him by the Greek contingent, as he lay forlornly but very visibly across a few flights of steps.

V
replenishing

This routine works brilliantly first thing in the morning, preferably every day:

❶ clean teeth (electric toothbrushes are best — ask any dentist)

note: avoid mirrors before cleaning if previous night had a red wine theme

❷ 2 glasses of water, ideally with liver tonic pills or powder (buy from health shop — see below)

❸ squeeze oranges for orange juice or eat orange

note: in the event of hangover, buy and drink copious amounts of crap-free fresh orange juice — one to two litres — works better than anything else

❹ eat more fruit, the more the better

❺ floss teeth, then rinse with mouthwash

Even a smoker will feel good after this. It's what the liver calls a perfect start to the day, ideally preceded or proceeded by exercise and/or sex (for mind and body).

The best alternatives to a fruit breakfast are fresh vegetable juice, wholemeal, multigrain or sourdough toast with vegemite or honey (it's okay to have some marg or preferably butter with toast, to prevent choking), muesli with soy milk or yoghurt, tomatoes and mushrooms and/or baked beans or other beans on toast, bacon on toast if you must eat dead animal. Things like sausages, eggs and bacon for breaky won't kill you; just steal your energy during lengthy digestion.

There are various liver tonic powders and pills available at health stores. You can either buy particular things which are super-good for the liver, such as milk thistle or slippery elm bark, or buy products which contain a mixture of liver-happy supplements. Pills/powder containing vitamins should ideally be taken with fruit or vegetable juice instead of water, because vitamins cannot be effectively consumed without tricking the body into thinking they're food. This goes for all vitamin supplements, so always have with food.

Are you coping with all this serious information? Can you keep the concentration up? Warning: more critical facts to follow. Get yourself a coffee or something more adult, jump up and down a few times, touch your toes. Wake up! You need to understand how the body works, so read on; focus. Try improving your posture.

Many drinkers hoe into greasy junk food if they wake up seedy, and consequently feel shithouse for the whole day. If you can't break this routine, try to at least have plenty of fruit juice first, or drink as much water as you can stomach.

Water is crucial for anyone at any time. For the serious drinker, it's our best defence. Mark and I are very fortunate to have a bush retreat where we can collect rainwater. Because gutters get mucky, we bought a water filter — a large attractive one with big filters that have to be changed a few times a year. It's liver heaven. The quality of the water you drink is going to affect your whole body and overall health. Your liver will be cleansed effectively and efficiently by high quality and pure drinking water. Strive for paranoidly obsessive water-quality control-freakdom.

When we were in the desert we bought all our water, spending a small fortune on it. Money well spent. Try keeping a huge container of good water by your bed and drink as much as possible before retiring/crashing, during the night or near morning. Get a potty if required. You may prefer to drink lots during the day, which is excellent. I'm hooked on tea, which is also healthy (standard or herb). Coffee addicts should abstain after about 4.00 pm and aim for only one or two per day. Personally, I'd rather save my liver for more fun pursuits than coffee.

I've heard from reputable sources that tea is also rich with caffeine. If so, why is it that after coffee I feel like I've been injected with amphetamines, whereas tea leaves me feeling normal and doesn't stop me sleeping? Plus tea has high antioxidant value. Maybe there's something tricky about the caffeine in tea that turns it into goodness. I wonder if the scientists could explain this, once they're over astronauts.

Finally, vitamins. Lots of beer ∞ lots of pissing ∞ loss of vitamins, particularly B and C, which are crucial for a healthy liver. As mentioned, always take a multi–B with food when you're in for a big session. Most days a multivitamin at lunchtime will suffice, maybe and/or an antioxidant with dinner. If a huge night is in store, take two milk thistle tablets before and after going out (with at least one glass of water) and two more in the morning. Slippery elm bark is also excellent (although someone told me there aren't too many slippery elms left, which leaves me concerned about my personal contribution to their demise).

There are many useful pills etc in health shops. Some of my favourites are: fish oil (cheap and very good for body), green tea (sensational for everything and boosts metabolism), chamomile and other herb teas (good anti–hangover weapon if drunk before, during or after wine), evening primrose oil and vitamin supplements designed to alleviate PMT for premenstrual women. Hopefully premenstrual men are already receiving professional attention.

If you're really serious about maximising health in

the long run, very effective vitamin pills are available. The long-term benefits of vitamin supplements are now scientifically proven and medically accepted. El Cheapo vitamins are like El Cheapo anything else. Results from independent scientific tests are useful when choosing the best vitamiun brands.

Are you still focusing? Do you need another drink? Not much more serious stuff to follow. Keep up the good work. You can do it!

Keeping well-hydrated is top priority for the healthy alcoholic. Important relevant facts:

- the body is made of mostly water (around 70%)

- only foods to have mainly water: fruit and vegetables (70% to 90%)

- all foods except fruit and vegetables need extra water for digestion (eg, carbohydrates, cheese, meat, junk foods and sweets)

- hangovers are due to dehydration

- fruit is much quicker to digest than any other food (30-45 minutes; compared to vegies 3 hrs, meat 8 hrs, eggs 24 hrs) and is best eaten on an empty stomach to take full advantage of the cleansing properties

- as well as being stomach and liver favourites, vegies and salad are crucial for body maintenance and repair

- green vegies are SuperVitamins (consume daily)

• ideal to have multi-coloured fruits and vegies to ensure a wide range of vitamins (not to mention flavour) — eg, orange, green, yellow, red

Occasionally you may misjudge, have a bad attitude or hard problem that needs drowning in alcohol → hangover, with depression. Top priority: forgive yourself and have mercy. Mollycoddle and spoil yourself. Watch telly/videos/DVDs all day and eat pizza and icecream (after the orange juice). If partner available, have as much sex as possible. Try hair of the dog. Relax. Be lazy. Take sickie and don't take guilt trip. Laugh at yourself. Don't listen to the judgmentalist in your head. Have a bath. Cook and eat. Enjoy going to bed early. "To err is human; to forgive, divine." Be divine!

VI
celebrate life, we're in it!

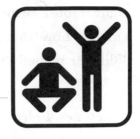

"Life's too short to muck around" — my teenage motto. The repercussions were fairly catastrophic in my youth. However, I still embrace the theme. For starters, it's true. Life is short, too short — so there's no time to waste. As my ex-hairdresser used to say (whilst making the most extraordinary alterations to my appearance, over a few champagnes):

"We're here for a good time, not for a long time."

In other words, life's here, this is it, let's go for it today! That may be why alcohol-free days (AFDs) are just not my thing. Once I tried one AFD per week, but my entire life became a stressful nightmare. I drank more on every other day of the week, due to panic.

For those with enough discipline to endure regular AFDs, go for it. No question it's good for your liver and whole body. But if you're like me, rest assured we're not alone, and it's healthier to enjoy it than to worry about it. This is a quotation from the Daily Mail, 17 October 1961:

I asked Madame Lily Bollinger, head of the Champagne House, who is in London to declare her 1955 Vintage, how she enjoyed her own product. Madame Bollinger replied thus:

"I drink it when I'm happy and when I'm sad. Sometimes I drink it when I'm alone. When I have company I consider it obligatory. I trifle with it if I'm not hungry and drink it when I am. Otherwise I never touch it — unless I'm thirsty."

You're not the only human who loves to drink, indulging daily. There are millions of us, and if there was less poverty in the world there would doubtless be billions more drinking enthusiasts.

Other animals get out of it too, like koalas on gum leaves, primates on fermenting fruit. Here in the Otways when the gum nuts are ripe, beautiful big gangangs soar around like drunken pilots. Nutcracking, they're approachable and unafraid; on the wing, reckless. Their flight is a wild dance, as they narrowly swerve bushes, trees, and human heads.

Birds don't like being told what to do, and nor do I. Have you ever met anyone who did? My eyes glaze over when anti-whatever preaching begins. But I do have accidental FAPs (fuck-all-piss days). These are great for the liver and don't stress the mind. My FAPs may be three cans/stubbies of beer. A couple of these in a row and I'm ready for anything (at least as far as I remember; it's a distant memory). You can work out your own quantities. For example, the amazing and youthful Winston Churchill drank a whole bottle of champagne every lunchtime and every dinner time (after a siesta, I believe). In between, he drank mainly straight spirits.

For Winston, an FAP would be spirits only, or a mere bottle of champers in a day! Like me, he avoided self-deprivation. What a great advertisement for the happy and healthy alcoholic he was. One night his housekeeper remarked, "You're drunk." His reply, "In the morning I'll be sober, but you'll still be ugly." From another perspective and on a different note, yet in keeping with the sentiment, Tom Waits;

"We're all gonna be just dirt in the ground."

Undeniable. Let's enjoy getting there! Embrace the present.

The author of this one is unknown:

"Imagine there is a bank which credits your account each morning with $86,400. It carries over no balance from day to day, allows you to keep no cash balance, and every evening cancels whatever part of the amount you had failed to use during the day.

"What would you do? Draw out every cent, of course! Well, everyone has such a bank. Its name is TIME. Every morning, it credits you with 86,400 seconds. Every night it writes off, as lost, whatever of this you have failed to invest to good purpose.

It carries over no balance. It allows no overdraft. Each day it opens a new account for you. Each night it burns the remains of the day. If you fail to use the day's deposits, the loss is yours. There is no going back. There is no drawing against the "tomorrow". You must live in the present on today's deposits. Invest it so as to get from it the utmost in health, happiness and success!

The clock is running. Make the most of today.

THE GIFT OF TIME.

To realize the value of ONE YEAR, ask a student who has failed a grade.

To realise the value of ONE MONTH, ask a mother who has given birth to a premature baby.

To realise the value of ONE WEEK, ask an editor of a weekly newspaper.

To realise the value of ONE DAY, ask a daily wage labourer who has kids to feed.

To realise the value of ONE HOUR, ask the lovers who are waiting to meet.

To realise the value of ONE MINUTE, ask a person who has missed the train.

To realise the value of ONE SECOND, ask a person who has avoided an accident.

To realise the value of ONE MILLISECOND, ask the person who has won a silver medal in the Olympics.

Treasure every moment that you have! And treasure it more because you shared it with someone special, special enough to have your time.

And remember time waits for no one.

Yesterday is history. Tomorrow a mystery.

Today is a gift. That's why it's called the present!"

VII
the importance of flossing

Don't worry, it's quick and easy!

If you have gum disease or plaque, bad semi-poisonous stuff is leaking into your body, through your stomach and liver (to the horror of both) which means the liver has to waste valuable energy filtering it.

Good oral hygiene will probably result in healthy gums and teeth that stay in for a lifetime.

Flossing is more important than cleaning with toothbrush.

Once a day is OK.

❶ clean (preferably with electronic toothbrush)

❷ floss, taking 1 to 2 minutes

❸ rinse/gargle with mouthwash

A well-looked-after mouth is a pleasure to kiss and be near. Bad breath is a result of poor oral hygiene

Avoid eating sugary things too often, and clean more when you do. If you eat real food — an abundance of fruit and vegies, proper bread, pasta and rice, nuts, legumes, seeds, garlic (especially raw), herbs, good olive oil; combined with not much butter, cheese, dead animal, junk, fried foods or sugary rubbish — your mouth will be happy, as will your stomach and liver, plus you'll look better.

Initially, I found flossing intolerably difficult. I was seriously worried that my fingers would fall off due to strangulation by floss, or my jaw permanently lock in an agonisingly open state. Then I bought these sort of enhanced flossers (available at chemists) which have handles — they should be called Finger Angels. After that, flossing became bearable. The best enhanced flossers are 3-D as opposed to 2-D; that is, like hooks, not just a V. It's a good way to start flossing.

Nowadays I'm so tough that I bravely floss with my fingers strangled and purple, jaw resolutely complying, but barely notice any discomfort and just enjoy having properly clean teeth and a nice mouth, with non-furry fangs. I'm not missing that ashtray-mouth sensation either; the smoker's wake-up call.

I'm trying to stop harassing my friends about the importance of flossing because it's a topic that few people are as passionate about as myself. But it's going to be impossible, until they're all diligent flossers too. It's just so crucial to good health, and if you'd prefer to have your own teeth in your mouth in later years, you must floss. If I don't make any progress with my friends in the next decade, maybe I'll try to meet lots of dentists. They understand the importance of flossing.

They also appreciate the huge difference a regular clean from a dental hygienist makes. If you can find a dentist who has an inhouse hygienist, for only a little more time and money you can transform your mouth into a heavenly bed of pearls. It may take a few visits, admittedly, if your starting point is a mouth full of multi-coloured slimy mystery mounds, but remember that diamonds were once coal.

Friends throw cynical glances when I explain that I love going to the dentist. Fillings and dental procedures can be terrifying and uncomfortable, if not downright painful, but if you floss daily and go to a hygienist every six months, you'll rarely need such intervention.

It's the feeling of perfectly clean smooth teeth that makes me look forward to getting a check-up and full clean. The hygienist cleans every tooth individually, using various means, and does a sterling job removing stains. You leave with whiter teeth, so you even look better. Plus it's cheaper than private dental cover in the long run.

You'd think my clear enthusiasm about all things dental would have friends sitting up, ears pricked, then rushing for the phone (to make an appointment). Astonishingly, they often prefer to cling to bad old habits, but they won't have much chance of clinging to their bad old teeth!

VIII
appearance matters

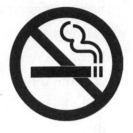

Whether or not appearance matters is something we could debate ad nauseam. Here I only wish to consider some matters of appearance based on personal observation.

• fruit is amazingly good for your skin, making it soft and shiny and smooth to touch

• give up smoking and your complexion will visibly improve in no time, plus your whole body will be softer to touch (due to oxygenation of previously starved cells), plus you won't stink and you'll be richer

• Vegetables are the Best Medicine: they heal your body. If you're sick, the more vegies you eat the better. Salad will give you an instant pickup. If you're injured, you need vegies. If it grows out of the earth, it's full of vitamins and youth-promoting antioxidants. Give your body a generous array and quantity of vegies and you will be rewarded, because all bodies are vegetable lovers.

• if anyone is game enough to take up one of the athletic forms of yoga, the benefits are phenomenal: it straightens the posture and makes you feel like you're getting younger; gives you great muscles and makes you strong; increases flexibility so that eventually the whole body moves with ease and grace; teaches balance and focuses the mind — a bit like trading your old bomb for a Rolls-Royce! (my yoga teacher looks like a Greek God)

• Rolls-Royces are not for everyone: the important point here is that any exercise will make you look better (and feel great)

• foods that tend to constipate are bad for everything, starting with your insides, and can eventually lead to obesity, gallstones, various forms of cancer (eg, stomach, bowel), plus will make you tired

• aloe vera is a miracle cure for burns, injuries and skin disorders; it's also great on the face and doesn't cost the earth, but it does come from the earth, not the chemical factory or science lab

• fresh air, getting close to nature and outdoor activities are more conducive to attractiveness than air-conditioning

• makeup clogs the pores, and high heels are bad for hips, back and skeleton generally

• men have higher muscle proportion than women so the need to exercise is even greater

• if your body moves easily and you're strong, it's got to be good for your sex life

• others are not obsessed by your appearance, only you

• the less you look in mirrors, the less you'll think about how you look (especially in a negative way)

• women are meant to have fat, and cellulite is natural and normal

• too much fat has negative health effects and can be associated with poor self-image; mobility is also affected, and the liver is overworked (sad but true).

Dieting is a pain and never works; too much deprivation. I've had a huge appetite ever since my grandmother began stuffing me with food as though her life depended on it (ie, from when I was zero) and she had many tricky ways to make us finish everything on the plate; "waste not, want not". I had a loose impression that if I didn't consume every last crumb, poor children in other countries would perish. Thus feeling like my stomach would explode became a virtue. Fortunately (for my grandmother) I rose to the occasion, and still heroically finish not only what's on my plate, but often anything else within reach.

However, I would never eat the same food combinations now — meat, vegies and bread (heaped with butter) "washed" down with fizzy drink, followed by dessert (eg, apple pie and ice cream) and tea and cake or biscuits. I think I'd expire instantly if I tried it these days, or at least wish I had expired.

Nowadays I'm comfortable with my appearance (most of the time) and enjoy not wearing makeup or following beauty regimes. I drink like a fish and eat hearty quantities of yummy food. Normally I'm bursting with energy and feel fantastic. You can do it too!

IX
master your metabolism

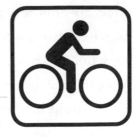

Having read (and experimented) enough about food to want to write this book, I know how to eat plenty but not be obese; a particularly impressive feat considering the calories of alcohol I consume daily. My usual is 3 or 4 beers (cans/stubbies), followed by a few glasses of wine, if not a bottle or more. Occasionally I'll get really serious. But I feel excellent most of the time, and look okay. Here's how to do it:

❶ EAT WELL: lots of fresh (preferably organic) fruit and vegies, nuts and seeds, healthy salad sandwiches and soups, different coloured fruits and vegies daily, pasta, rice, good quality olive oil, garlic, chilli, ginger (sometimes raw), herbs, spices, beans, tofu, soy milk

❷ WATER: very good quality water (preferably with liver tonic) in morning, more water during night, tea during day (standard and herb)

❸ EXERCISE: my own preferences are swimming, walking and yoga. Swimming is perfect for aerobic stimulation and metabolism boosting; very good weight control tool. Walking is relaxing and easy; even three 20-minute walks per week is way better than no exercise. Yoga is a miracle and has put me in touch with my whole body, inside and out. But it's not for everyone. Iyengar Yoga is very physically demanding. I started at 33. It would be ideal to start younger.

It takes quite a lot of exercise to keep me in shape, due to generous alcohol and food intake. My aim is to swim and practise yoga twice weekly, usually exercising for about an hour. I might go for a walk as well, or instead, leaving two or three days free for body relaxation and muscle recuperation. I frequently miss out on swimming or yoga practice, because I don't feel like it or it's inconvenient. If your body is tired or you're not in the mood, be lazy. But if sloth becomes the Norm, so will you.

Any exercise is great for your physical and psychological health: eg, tennis, sex, footy, dancing, jogging, bush walking, squash, aerobics, gym, cycling, walking, swimming, self-defence, martial arts, athletics, basketball and netball, cricket, pilates.

This is getting a bit serious again, eh? Yes, exactly. It is serious! Not understanding your metabolism is like not knowing how to drive your car, only worse (because you're not trapped in your car for life).

Getting your metabolism going by exercising 3 to 5 days per week will make you energetic, fit and healthy, while improving your appearance, posture and mental agility. The ball's in your court.

Eating also stimulates the metabolism. That's why you'll be healthier if you eat breakfast. If you don't, your body is in go-slow starvation mode from the start of the day and you'll reserve calories rather than burn them. Lunch is important for the same reason, although the liquid amber option is tempting on weekends, which might lead to metabolic shutdown if taken too far.

Exercising at the start of the day is a perfect metabolism kick-start and improves your mood and energy levels for the whole day. Alternatively, any exercise that follows food will aid digestion, increase the metabolic rate and prevent weight gain.

After eating, leave 30 to 60 minutes before easy exercises such as walking; 2 to 3 hours after a big meal or before serious exercise such as squash or running. If you exercise enough to promote sweating and a bit of heavy breathing, you've achieved the objective of increasing your metabolic rate.

Aerobic exercise is fantastic because it makes the blood race around the body, distributing oxygen and stimulating everything. Good also for detoxing. The best bit is that once you start doing any regular exercise, you feel extra good, which is an incentive to keep it up.

How many people do you know who enthusiastically take up some new fitness regime, like going to the gym or jogging, and boast that they love it so much they're doing it five or more days a week, followed months later by the inevitable complete loss of interest due to boredom and overexposure, plus the realisation that there's more to life than exercise?

There's a message here. Just like strict diets, it won't last. Much wiser to be moderate. Start by exercising three times a week and be content with that. Don't do exactly the same thing too many times a week or put pressure on yourself about doing X amount of exercise every week. If you make rules, you'll only break them, then plunge into a sea of guilt.

Let your body and mood dictate what and how much you do. If you don't really feel like doing it, don't. Sometimes you may want to have more than the usual number of consecutive lazy days. No worries. Your body loves a break now and then. You don't want to be an ob-sessed exercise fanatic. The aim is for exercise to become a normal part of life, on an ongoing long-term basis.

Choose activities you know you'll enjoy once you get going. There's no need to exhaust yourself repeatedly, or you may start to dread it. Do as much as you feel like doing each time, without putting great expectations on yourself before starting. Just focus on getting going and then let your body dictate how long and hard you do it.

So if gym or jogging, swimming, aerobics etc appeals to you, don't be an instant junkie. Try two or three days a week for a few months, maybe complemented by another form of exercise on another day (eg, walking). Embrace too much at once and your passion may expire with equal rapidity (because sadly, like everything, honeymoons end). If you gradually build up to exercising four or five days a week, it's more likely to become an integrated and natural part of your lifestyle.

Exercise speeds up grog metabolisation, because your body works harder. Thus if you exercise and drink simultaneously, you can drink even more. If balance is visibly impeded, however, or stumbling, fumbling and colliding unintentionally with the ball replace your usual athletic prowess, sport should cease. But as you can't play tennis, cricket, football or much else with a can, stubbie or wine glass in hand, the necessity of putting your drink down results in slower consumption. It's a total health kick. Just remember to supplement usual liquid intake with water if you're exercising hard enough to sweat.

Typically, the classy and wine-loving French invented boulles; the one sport that not only tolerates inebriation but practically demands it. Sober people should only be permitted to partake if they're under about 10 (ie, too young to be any good) or seriously lack athleticism and ball skills (eg, computer nerds) or if they want to umpire, serve drinks or play standby nurse (gay men are the best).

X
get your timing right

We're frequently advised to have a huge breaky, big lunch and small dinner, plus to never drink on an empty stomach. If that works for you, go for it. Sounds great for weight control. Because I love food and always look forward to dinner, being the fun work-is-over part of the day, my routine is the opposite:

• water then fruit for breaky

• cups of tea during morning

• salad or vegie rich lunch (eg, salad sandwiches, pasta, soup, tofu — anything with vegies) OR beer if it's the weekend; lunch can wait!

• 2-3 beers after work, always on an empty stomach

• at least plan to start preparing food and drinking wine simultaneously; very good for the digestion to have food and wine together, plus enhances chance of not getting blotto

• failing the above, drink wine — probably too much — followed by massive and unsophisticated pig-out, then sudden uninvited crash-out (snoring in chair in contorted state)

EVEN WHEN this happens I'll be fine the next day if dinner was healthy and hearty, with water consumed during night, being too full and buggered to fit it in before staggering to bed, especially now that Mark refuses to carry me, muttering about bad backs or something (what happened to Death Before Dishonour? If it's good enough for the squash court...).

You probably have eating and drinking patterns that you enjoy and don't want to change. But if you know your health is suffering, remember that when you eat you make a choice between food that will be loved by your body and food that will make you tired (and probably fat, which isn't ideal). Getting used to healthy eating is not much harder than trying it. "You are what you eat."

Spirits are spooky. It's so tricky getting the timing right. It's hard to tell when you've had too much. Collapsing after attempting a vertical position is a sure sign; but the unicorn has bolted. Many spirit lovers suffer next day. Combining spirits with cola or other sugary junk is very tough on stomach and liver. Best chance of staying in good health if you're a big spirits drinker is to have water at the same time, and always eat. Try mixing with water instead of cola.

Spirits-induced hangovers are serious. Beer, cider,

stout/Guinness are the most forgiving. Champagne is pretty good (I guess it's the bubbles). Wine is fine if not drunk too quickly, and red is safer. Fortified wines (port, muscat etc) are OK if consumed slowly. Fluorescent sugary teenage drinks are tragic from any angle.

There was a time, thankfully long past, when Mark and I indulged heavily in fortifieds, buying yummy cheapish stuff in refillable litre bottles. The first half bottle tended to go down sensibly, if not with cultured elegance, after which all hell broke loose. A litre of port packs a punch, and is an exceptionally effective painkiller. Thank God for that, because the number of dreadful accidents I endured during the fortified years were extraordinary.

Once I burnt half the skin off my forearm after tripping on a stump while carrying the gas lantern. It took a while to convince Mark that I may have sustained a real injury. He thought I had a few prickly tea tree scratches. Suffice to say one look and he knew better. When my sister saw it at work a few days later, she screamed. I still have scars from that one and, more relevantly, these days I'm scared of fortifieds. None-theless, I do have friends who live on them and manage to pace themselves appropriately. That's the key; pace. Bit like sex really.

It's a good idea to check the time when you get yourself a new drink, to guard against accidental skolling.

Sometimes when Mark and I are at Carlisle River we'll drink for more or less the whole day by just doing it slowly: 1 beer every 45 minutes to 1 hour, or two wines per hour. This is plausible if we're active — eg, gardening — but sooner or later the pixies set in. Pixies are miniature alcoholics who live in wine glasses and bottles of wine and spirits. They have a lot to answer for. If the wine in your bottles evaporates with inexplicable rapidity, you've got pixies too.

When you drink slowly the pixies are trapped in bottles and cans, plus your body has a chance to metabolise or digest the alcohol and the liver isn't over-whelmed. Snacking is very wise, to keep your stomach happy and you grounded. Fast drinking is a fast route to bed, with no root when you get there!

XI
genes and gender

What's in your jeans is important because men tend to be heavier, hence have more blood in which to process the alcohol. Although personally I can drink most men under the table, many women are not so lucky. If you're skinny — be it male or female — you don't have many fat cells in which to store alcohol and not that much blood in which to disperse it, so chances are you're frequently first under the table. Some thin people may find light alcohol keeps them on their feet longer. Others with very fast metabolisms seem quite able to keep up with the cuddliest of us.

Maybe because of their genes. I'm very grateful to my forebears for evolving their livers so brilliantly, and I'm a believer in exercising the liver. The medical profession don't seem to have embraced this concept. This worries me not. It's hard to take them too seriously when they were even more embarrassing than me in the uni tavern. So although, admittedly, I can cite no authority as yet, I remain convinced that the drinking my parents and grandparents engaged in has led to the development of tough and resilient livers that will rise to the occasion, certainly if/when treated with respect. Mine gets a good dose of TLC and the food it loves, as well as the alcohol. I feel great. So if I'm killing myself, it's fun dying.

If, like my partner Mark, your forebears are/were teetotallers, just bear it in mind. Be realistic. Experiment. Listen to your body. It speaks very loudly. Here are a few clues about body talk:

• regularity is a sign of good health and constipation is not

• yellow eyes reflect a tired liver

• cracking and redness at the corners of the mouth mean you've had too much alcohol and not enough food, resulting in B-vitamin deficiency (vitamin B cream fixes it quickly and can be used as a preventive measure)

• pale translucent eyes reflect a lack of vitamins and nutrients

• belching results from indigestion (overloaded stomach)

• if your stomach is full, it doesn't want any more and will have to stockpile anything extra for later (like too much in the in-tray)

• headaches may result from dehydration and/or smoking

• not sleeping well could be caused by too much caffeine or stress and worry, or too much pizza, ice cream, chocolate etc

• a bad hangover means you've overdone it (think of it as a learning experience and make the most of the day you have)

• if your body feels great, it's probably in great shape

• inactivity breeds laziness; exercise is energising

• increase your metabolism and you can do more and eat more and drink more

• practice works: try it with exercise (the muscles have memory); drinking (the liver learns); chilli (the taste buds adjust); sex (even those muscles improve); healthy food (gets yummier)

• shower your body in love and care, not criticism, and you'll get along well with yourself; remembering your body — or at least hopefully most of it — is with you for your whole life (although I once heard a radio show about people looking forward to gradually exchanging all their natural body parts for man-made replacement bits, including a sort of computer brain, so that they could live for a very long time — they were rich Americans, of course)

• when you give your stomach healthy and useful

food, it's like belly bliss; so coping with all that alcohol isn't too hard.

Aim to discover the right balance for you.

You are, after all, unique.

XII
food and cooking

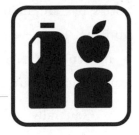

If you're not into cooking, are you sure you're drinking enough? You need the appropriate accompaniments: wine, music, cute apron, dance floor just in case. Maybe you haven't embraced the kitchen but you're lucky enough to live with someone who has, or rich enough to eat out well — and "well" means fresh and healthily prepared. If, like me, you love cooking — or even just enjoy it sometimes — here are some easy ways to make the most of the food you prepare, in order to gain maximum goodness from it.

Aside from taking a keen interest in articles on food and health in magazines, press, radio etc over the years, I've read a few helpful books on the subject: "The Good Food Book" by Des Buchhorn BSc ND; "Fit For Life" by Harvey and Marilyn Diamond; "The Liver Cleansing Diet" by Dr Sandra Cabot MD; "The Healthy Liver & Bowel Book" by Dr Sandra Cabot MD.

Unlike the learned authors above, I have nothing more than a BA, bachelor of arts, although I clearly deserve a bachelor of alcoholism as well. Studying such books has taught me so much about food/body/digestion that I'm near saturation point and have little desire to incorporate one more fact or theory. But you won't learn much about drinking from these books.

Generally they insist it's tragically harmful and you've got serious problems if you drink more than two drinks per day for women, four drinks per day for men, stressing the importance of alcohol-free-days (AFDs) and so on and so on, until it's a wonder a pisspot like me is alive at all. Clearly my FAP concept is ahead of its time. How much more user-friendly, not to mention ic-friendly, is the fuck-all-piss day?

I don't feel like I'm about to drop off my perch or get sick, develop liver cancer or suffer the ghastly side-effects of drinking as described in health books. I'm fit, energetic, very rarely get sick. A good friend of mine, also a daily drinker, reckons he never gets the colds and flu's endured by the masses. He puts it down to the grog wiping out the germs! My experience is adding weight to his theory.

It's due to experience and experiments on my own body over the years that I'm keen to help other drinkers get healthy. Also, unhealthy drinkers feed a stereotypical image in society that alcoholics are hopeless, jobless slobs etc. It's a bullshit myth. The majority of big drinkers I've met are intelligent people with responsible jobs. So they drink heavily. Big deal. Many people are addicted to headache pills and painkillers, sweet foods or dieting, even whinging. Would you rather be one of them?

We need a Revolutionary Drinkers Party or Free To Drink campaign. It's time to stop being ashamed and giving yourself a hard time for drinking what someone else says is "too much". It's your body and your life, and you've only got one of each. Ditch the guilt trips and New Year's resolutions. Have a Personal Revolution instead. I describe myself as an alcoholic, quite proudly. Why not call a spade a spade? It's so much easier to understand a spade that way. If you're trying to convince yourself it's a hammer, you'll be fighting with it forever. If you admit it's a spade, you can do so many useful things with it. Just like with yourself: you can be a happy, healthy alcoholic if you choose.

Time again for serious concentration, so get yourself ready and then study on!

Firstly, it's important to understand digestion. As already mentioned, fruit digests exceptionally quickly and is therefore best eaten before other food; otherwise it gets stuck in the queue and goes off before evacuating, instead of giving you a thorough clean on the inside. Next easiest and healthiest food to digest is vegetables, the more the merrier, and great to have a variety of colours.

Secondly, try not to combine too many different

food types at one time. If you're in weight-conscious mode, have vegies with meat OR cheese OR pasta OR rice OR fish OR bread OR beans, rather than mix these up. It's also good and very yummy to have vegies with pasta and cheese OR with bread and meat etc. The most important thing is to have the vegies.

Salad, being raw, is even more packed with vitamins and antioxidants. As long as it's not smothered in mayonnaise or similar, salad is about as healthy as it gets. Avocado is very good in salad; eg, with lettuce, carrot, bean sprouts, spring onions. Tabouli and/or salad and avocado sandwiches are excellent. Humus and/or mustard are also delicious in salad sandwiches, as is pesto.

If you're a big bloke with a big appetite and you're not worried about a cuddly beer gut (like my man), the thought of a salad sandwich for lunch fills you with horror, culminating in a bolt to the pie shop. But the salad sandwich intolerant can still try to think in terms of proportions. Ideally, make sure the vegetable portion is (1) there and (2) makes up a third or more of the quantity. Rice and pasta are very good for satisfying a big appetite, combined with meat or seafood or beans and vegies. But don't add cheese.

Deep fried is liver misery, so you're better off with a hamburger than fish and chips. Batter is not good, unless purchased in an expensive restaurant where all food is art and the female customers are on diets anyway.

Not to mention the waiters.

But skinny chefs — what's going on there? Eating disorders, not enough taste-testing? Not to be trusted.

Eggs — now, they'd make excellent politicians. Difficult and very time-consuming to digest, promote excess burping and wind, often foul smelling at the end of the line. Best taken only in moderation, combined with something easier on the enzymes.

Nuts — extra good, but too many can be hazardous. I adore nuts. Sometimes I find them irresistibly morish, and OD, resulting in some pretty bad shit (literally). Buying small quantities means a chance of controlling the nut munchies. Best not eaten after or with other food (unless adding sensible quantities to vegie-based meals, for flavour and crunch). But there's usually too many for the dish, and the rest are barely worth storing and might go stale... (chomp chomp).

Bread — if you choose wholemeal, sourdough, rye, multigrain and other healthy types of bread, and eliminate or minimise butter or margarine, any sort of sandwich that includes salad is happy body food.

In the event of abysmal food combining and subsequent stomach over-expansion, don't despair! Remember, antacids or liver salts taken an hour or two after the feast will help. A walk is ideal, if you have the strength to lift your enlarged body off the couch/floor.

Wine helps keep the digestive enzymes going, plus enhances the likelihood of losing consciousness, which will at least stop you from worrying about which clothes will fit tomorrow.

A walk next morning will get your stomach working and should restore your self-respect. If you want to feel saint-like, only have a couple of oranges or orange juice for breakfast. If you're furious with yourself and nothing short of punishment is sufficient, have only fruit for lunch as well and you'll be skinny and ravenous by teatime.

This can easily backfire, either because you're starving or because your super-ego has gone to town and won the day, but your suppressed child is ripe for rebellion, with the whole over-eating routine beginning afresh. It's better to relax and take a few days to get back to normal size after a day or two of gluttony.

Infuriatingly, it takes me weeks or months to rediscover my wardrobe-friendly size after weeks of holiday wining and dining.

Moving on to some food facts…

❶ Deep Fried

Unless you're a hermit (in which case I should commend the distributors) you've heard that deep fried foods are not good for you. It's true. They're very fatty and fattening, with most of the nutrients long deceased (if they ever existed). The oil has been cooked too long or too high and hence its chemical structure has altered so that even if it was a healthy oil to begin with, it has been ruined and is now rancid. This mutated oil is a problem for your stomach and liver, and has nothing beneficial left in it.

My doctor once suggested to me that beer wasn't likely to do much harm, aside from being useless calories. I no doubt replied it wasn't useless; it's my anti-stress missile. I've told him all about my drinking, but I have a suspicion he thinks I'm exaggerating, because I don't look appalling. Maybe he's an old hippy like me, and doesn't believe in only science.

We need to bring the hippies back. Just look at what they've done to the world since we went underground. The next revolution will have to be led by the rich; those of us lucky enough to afford good wine.

❷ The Good Oil

Quality oils come in many flavours: olive, macadamia, walnut, sesame, grape seed — all excellent foods and yummy if not overheated. That's the important bit. You'll be doing not only your liver a favour by taking this into account when cooking or buying food; the flavour of the oil comes through beautifully when cooked gently or added at the end.

So how to heat up onions and garlic, for example?

Instead of heating oil in the pan, use water, stock, tomato puree, juice or wine; bring to light bubbling point and add chopped onions. The slower and longer you cook the onion, the better. It reduces to a yummier and yummier flavoursome base for any dish, and caramelises beautifully. Use plenty of onions. You can do the same with carrots or eggplant.

Don't add garlic too early; it's more potent when added later. If you crush the garlic it maximises aroma, flavour and medicinal values. Think of garlic as a detox tool, and blast it through your system like a cleaning agent. It helps cheese digest. A "garlic bomb" of parmesan cheese and raw garlic gives your mouth and sinuses a sensational blast. All garlic and cheese combinations are good. Raw garlic is loved by your body. True friends will get over it.

Other great flavoursome body-cleansers include chilli, ginger, balsamic vinegar, mustard. These are perfect for flavouring your dish: add to onion any time. Always taste-test to get quantities right (but try not to taste-test the entire dish before serving).

Chilli, like friends, should be treated with both love and respect. One night my grandmother rang when I was cooking dinner. Mark's got this funny idea that we're always on the phone for hours, so he helpfully took over the preparations and continued with the chilli chopping. An hour later my phone call had finished and

Mark was on the floor in a foetal position, after relieving himself, suffering from what I can only describe as "chilli dick". Judging from the degree and duration of agony he endured, it was even worse than "chilli eye". No sex that night.

Less dangerous are anchovies, which give an excellent fishy/salty taste to the onion base for extra bite. Honey added is delicious. Also good are tamari, spices, herbs, curry, turmeric. It's easy to make your water-based (or other non-oil-based) "frying start" very yummy without oil. But add as much oil as you like later on, taste-testing as you go. You won't need as much because the flavour is fuller when not overheated.

So add oil late rather than early, to a gently simmering dish and never let it bubble furiously. Always taste-test, adding salt and pepper if desired towards the end. Too much salt or pepper can ruin a cooking creation. Heartbreaking. Too much taste-testing can ruin an appetite, but not if the food is sensational.

An easy and yummy way to have toast is with olive oil and balsamic vinegar, instead of margarine or butter. It's a healthy quick meal if the bread is good. If you have no vegies and no time, you can still have useful food by including something nutricious: vegemite (yeast and B vitamins); honey (sugar energy and good for eyes and mood); grainy bread; canned tomatoes or tomato soup.

Some foods-in-cans are still very good for you.

These include (fortunately) canned tomatoes, and red salmon (but increase in salmon farming is leading to more fatty salmon that can't exercise because of over-crowding and have to be fumigated with chemicals due to the sewerage they create etc, so let's hope John West rejects these ones!).

Canned tomatoes make a fantastic base for any-thing, best cooked gently for ages, letting them reduce and intensify, resulting in a beautiful rich flavour. The same slow frying that works perfectly with onions and tomatoes (canned or otherwise) is equally effective with carrots or chard stalks. The green chard leaves should be added near the end of cooking.

Onions can be combined with tomatoes, carrots or chards. With or without other flavours introduced as it simmers gently, it's an easy way to get soups, pasta sauces, vegetable, tofu or meat dishes off to a great start. If you're only adding sausages, seafood or meat to the base (low water content foods) the onions etc will eventual-ly brown to perfection and you'll wish there were mountains more (especially if you've fallen victim to over-exuberant taste-testing).

❸ Pasta, Bread Etc

Excellent. Potentially "bloating" if, like myself, your stomach is a bottomless pit when it comes to bread, pasta, potatoes or rice. Best way of preventing this is eat-ing slowly — nothing short of impossible usually. I find it easier (plus it's healthier) to accompany these great texture foods with lots of vegies, or at least pesto or something with goodness in it.

If you have your pasta etc with large quantities of meat or cheese, it's tough on the stomach enzymes. Keep the quantities moderate and it's not too bad. Seafood is easier to digest and a bit lighter, plus contains many nutrients the body thrives on. But vegies are what your body needs most.

Rice tends to expand, sometimes to an alarming degree, in the stomach. Occasionally I have nearly exploded due to rice gluttony. It's horrendous, because it can take days to recover, during which time food can't be enjoyed with the usual fervour, or at least not without a noticeable increase in overall size. But rice is a good food, if you're a self-controlled type (bit rare amongst ics). A delicious and nutrient-rich variety is wild rice, which is multicoloured and extra chewy.

Rice shouldn't be reheated unless it's been fully cooled down in fridge after initial cooking, as warm rice is conducive to bacterial activity. Lastly, as usual, wholegrain is more nutritious, and if you shop right it's also more delicious.

XIII
shit happens

There are dangerous traps a drinker may fall into. I've already confessed to suffering fairly bad injuries while pissed. I certainly wouldn't drink and drive. I do drink and passenger, for the fun factor. I've heard it's illegal, but find it hard to take laws seriously when they're ludicrous. Turning now to sense (which contrary to popular belief is rare, not common), let's bravely focus on alcoholic negatives.

❶ Brain

Last night, I have been informed, I was in bed hours before dark, presumably blotto. I remember cooking and eating very yummy home-grown food —broccoli and fetta entrée, pesto pasta with spinach, not to mention wild flying parmie characteristically targeting my mouth. A pre-food riesling set the early afternoon off to a frivolous start, cemented by the with-food chardonnay and finally wiped out completely by the know-it's-naughty-but-who-cares third bottle of white.

That third bottle has not registered in my memory chip, and to be frank, I suspect that particular chip is in less than mint condition. My suspicion is based on strange next-morning discoveries of things like condoms next to bed, with no actual memory of sex; a multitude of bread crumbs scattered in munching zones, or parmesan bits, but no recollection of eating (grateful, however, that eating did occur, because stomach is full instead of sick). Plus if I say to Mark something like, "Who won the cricket?" he looks at me as though a stupider person never walked the earth. Really, he should be used to it by now.

I am. It's not ideal, admittedly, but shit happens. And not just to drinkers but in all walks of life: shit happens and it's something we may as well accept. So I suffer short-term memory loss at times. Yes, this is true. The way I see it, an excess of mindboggling brain cells has been my lot for long enough. It's not so much brain cell death, as brain cell culling.

❷ Body

Then there's my appearance. Would definitely look better if didn't drink. Would also be bored.

Many years ago (at 23 and already a good drinker) I went alcohol-free for seven weeks, inspired by some ghastly embarrassing incident which, mercifully, I have since forgotten.

Life was very different on the wagon. Days were long and I didn't need much sleep. Socialising and partying became uninteresting. Work was more enjoyable, because not-at-work had lost its celebratory character. I looked great and my figure improved, leading to vanity. My attention focused more on my appearance, as though the possibility of beauty made looks more important. I was surprised by this reaction and didn't like it. Vanity is so hollow.

My mind was crystal clear. My mood didn't vary much. I was perfectly in control and even started to feel a bit condescending towards other more frivolous viewers. I enjoyed the extreme clarity for quite a while and was convinced I'd never return to anything close to daily drinking because I liked being in such great condition.

As time went on, boredom crept in. There was no excitement, no challenge, as if all days were the same. The thought of having a drink entered my mind and filled me with stress and excitement. I was by now quite obsessed by my exceptional physical health; hence the stress and fear of loss of control.

The day came when I decided to relax and have a few drinks. I was totally excited, like a kid before a birthday party, and secretly annoyed that my friends didn't share the sense of occasion. They were used to drinking so remained quite calm at the thought of going to the pub for a few beers and eight ball. I was high at the mere thought.

Pretending to be calm, I drank at the pub like everyone else, and my anticipation was nothing compared to the actual experience of creeping inebriation.

It was exhilarating. I loved the effect it had on my mood/state of mind/reality — it was so much fun! I felt like devoting myself to partying and never fully returning to the control-freak state I'd been immersed in. To my disappointment, my friends were content to drink sensibly rather than go overboard that night.

I've never looked back. For the next few weeks I was over-excited by alcohol, but soon returned to my usual consumption levels and imperfect appearance, happily shedding the vanity. I'll never forget how uplifting that first drink was after such abstinence — a period loved more by my liver than my mind. I'd even like to do it again one day, but the decades are rolling on and I just haven't been in the mood.

❸ Money

It can be expensive to drink in style. Like most fledgling drinkers, I was less than stylish in my early drinking years. These days I insist on reasonable quality wines because the real cheapies make me feel sick. They're hangover material. Same goes for crappy spirits. Better to treat your body with respect as you mature, so that you age like a good wine rather than merely ferment. Your body is your earthly vehicle and has already got you this far. Give it a break. It thrives on quality.

❹ Heat

I was just racking my brain about more disadvantages of drinking when I remembered the heat issue. I'm hot. Not all drinkers are hot, but many of us are. It's because the body has to work harder to deal with the alcohol. In my case, I had a tendency to get hot even before I discovered drinking, and would go red in the face after not much exercise. People with different metabolisms will react differently, but an increase in body temperature and a bit of face reddening is common.

Going suddenly very red could be an allergic reaction to a certain food or drink (or the chemicals in it) or drinking too quickly. If you've been skolling, the cure is obvious. Red faces can also be caused by stress or sudden embarrassment, which may or may not be easily overcome.

Being hot is something I'm accustomed to. Most of my clothes are sleeveless, and wet hair in summer is super-cooling. It's annoying if I get suddenly hot and can't cool down, especially if it's somewhere I don't want to be, like in one of those airconditioned buildings that could double as a pizza oven, but worrying about or focusing upon it is pointless. If your head is full of worry or fury about something, try changing the topic. You can choose what you focus on.

By not only drinking to my heart's content but also eating and exercising a lot, I keep my metabolism at a fast rate and this creates heat. People comment, "Aren't you cold?" because of my summery attire. Sometimes I react internally with aggression and wish I could punch them, then hesitate long enough to regain my socially-conditioned composure and say something like, "No, just feel my shoulder," invariably impressing them with my warmth. The alternative reply, "I'm always hot," leaves them squirming, not knowing whether to inquire as to my state of health or escape immediately from a nymphomaniac. One friend took the bait and responded, "Oh Cindy, I don't know how Mark keeps up."

You may have a different physical issue that you suspect relates to alcohol consumption. This is a multiple choice question. Do you:

(a) give up drinking immediately

(b) keep drinking but whinge about your "problem"

(c) try to give up drinking but fail repeatedly and hate yourself for it

(d) get used to it and stop calling it a problem.

Actually, the answer is so obvious that there really was no choice.

❺ Time

Drinking occupies a good deal of my time. This is my preference, because when I'm drinking I'm happy. Feeling good each morning also means getting enough sleep, the amount of which needs to be balanced with the previous day's consumption. If there's a hangover looming, better to sleep through it. I would spend more of my life awake if I didn't drink. This doesn't bother me, but some may see it as a negative.

In the latter part of the day when I'm likely to be under the influence to a greater or lesser extent, the chances of performing tasks that require intense concentration or precision are minimised, due to lack of coordination and the competing attraction of leisurely pursuits like talking, cooking, gardening, dancing, sex, eating — having a generally good time in whatever situation. Wandering around listening to music can be a perfect pastime.

I adore dancing and can't get enough of it. It's such a celebration of life, expressive and exhilarating. I've been in raptures since rediscovering Neil Dia-mond's classic live album Hot August Night. Dancing to inspiring music all over my bush pad — perfect.

Just remember, Safety First. For example, after two to three beers Mark might do lawnmowing or wood chopping, but not tree-felling or chainsaw work. I might chop vegies or fence baby trees, but wouldn't do yoga or hammer in nails. Fortunately for my fingers and my career, I rarely hammer nails. I got plenty of practice when Mark and I were building our house in the bush; never quite mastered it.

We began and ended our building days as amateurs, but managed to build most of a quite classy mudbrick house. Like all owner-built houses, it will never be finished. A professional builder has taken over. Last time I saw Andrew, he said he'd be back on Monday. That was years ago. Things like time are different in the bush.

Building memories are great, and often filled with tinnies. When Mark and I were "helping" with the roof, Andrew (the builder of few words but many VBs) said to Mark, "Knock a few nails in those." "Sure," Mark replied, thrilled to be more than a useless onlooker (a role I merrily embraced, plus making sure we all had enough tinnies). Mark proceeded to hammer six-inch nails into lengths of wood that were laid out in very particular fashion on the floor.

After some time (because it takes considerable effort to get those mothers in) Andrew came along and, without speaking, yanked out the nails. He then did a bit of extra-efficient nailing himself, not the least impressive part of which was that he nailed the tilt-up wooden roof structure together, instead of into the floor as Mark had done!

But Mark and I were brilliant mudbrick layers, yet another task well suited to a tinnie or two (which is Australian for too many to count). When we spent four long weekends making render by the traditional Japanese method of painfully handsieving every bit of a massive quantity of muddy stuff repeatedly through wire mesh in a wheelbarrow until it turned into perfectly smooth apricot coloured render, drinking was essential.

Don't pretend you're stone cold sober when you're not. If you're not afraid to call yourself a drinker, you can get realistic about how much you really drink and the effect it has upon you. Count drinks, look at the time, monitor your own physical and mental response. The great thing about drinking is that it always works; ie, gets you tipsy and eventually pissed. Most other drugs become less effective as time goes on and hence the addict needs more and more. With drinking it's quite easy to work out, through realistic self-analysis, how much is too much and how fast is too fast. Admittedly it takes a while, but the experiments are very amusing. You can rest assured that others will remember the really embarrassing bits if you forget them.

Some constructive activities make great drinking partners, like gardening. Enjoying yourself by singing or any form of artistic expression is excellent therapy and a great way to spend time. With or without a drink in hand, activities that require physical and/or mental stimulation are the most rewarding.

I would have lost my sanity at Marla Travellers Rest, working so hard on the land rights case in the desert, if it wasn't for dancing. Around midnight I'd be dancing with great enthusiasm, earplugs in, alone in my room or while Mark snored in bed. Usually I'd be near naked and would admire myself in the mirror (looking great in the darkness) as I danced like crazy, my body desperate for movement and my mind for release. Every second was rejuvenating. Tired though I was, the dancing was as crucial as sleep.

How my father Deane and all the others involved kept their sanity, or even if they did, remains a mystery. Physical exhaustion is nothing compared to losing it mentally. While dancing I'd be smiling and laughing at myself, enlivening the body while relaxing the mind. Then I could sleep well and wake up happy. Much better than going to bed with a head full of work and worry, panicking about how little sleep was possible and waking up in the same anxious state.

Exercise will give you more energy than extra sleep. Dragging yourself out of bed early enough to exercise before work is an effort worth making. You'll be physically and mentally switched on all day. You don't need to spend much time exercising to get big rewards.

Becoming obsessed with exercise is stressful, like any obsession, and tedious for your lifestyle and your friends. Balance the pleasure (eg, drinking) with body maintenance (exercise, good food) and you can enjoy the best of all worlds.

A day spent with friends, talking and drinking, can be viewed as wasted (and some may well get wasted) or it can be treasured as a celebration of friendship and life, filled with laughter and great memories. For the drinker, some days may start with huge plans and finish with premature loss of consciousness. The next day you choose whether to call this a waste of time or an abundance of naughty fun.

❻ Embarrassing events

All drinkers have done stupid and embarrassing things at times. So have all humans. You'd have to be pretty up yourself to think that others actually care about your occasional misdemeanours. Focusing endlessly on mistakes you make is counterproductive. Grow up and get over it. Unless you've injured another person, physically or mentally, and need to make amends with that person, move on. You'll achieve nothing by torturing yourself with bouts of self-criticism and heavy judgments. Nothing will change the past. You can easily get yourself into a state of complete misery. You can even spread your misery around, but nothing is achieved. Well, except you'll be miserable.

Let's take some examples. You get pissed too quickly and vomit in front of the in-laws. You fall over in clumsy fashion. You have sex with the wrong person and wish you hadn't. You wet the bed. You wake up with don't-know-who and who-knows-where. You fart loudly while laughing too hard in toffy company. You get uncontrollable hiccups. You tell your least favourite relative what you really think of them. You flirt outrageously with the boss. You gossip mercilessly. One way or another, you humiliate yourself.

Gee, that's pretty earth-shattering.

XIV
shit matters

Despite overuse of the expletive, most people shy away from talking about shit in all its forms, and consequently the world is full of people who know almost nothing about it. There are those who are full of shit and don't know it, those who eat shit, those whose lives are shit, those who are oblivious to shit in the world around them. Worse still, there are those who don't give a shit.

At the most fundamental level, too few people understand the significance of the shit they quickly hide by flushing the toilet. Many are au fait with dream interpretation, but few with shit interpretation. If you're in the shit-scared majority, stop abolishing your natural bodily excrement so quickly to the hidden wonders of the sewerage system and enormity of the oceans. Your shit tells a story and it's an important one. It's the tale of how your body is dealing with what you're dishing up. You need to study it.

Mark and I were toilet-free for at least 10 years in the bush, so for three days a week it was impossible not to view one's shit. It had to be seen to be buried. This is how I stumbled upon (metaphorically speaking) the importance of studying it. After a while it's easy to relate output to input. Soon the relationship between good shit and good food becomes clear.

Another player is our favourite demon. If you combine lots of alcohol with not much food, your stomach will be awash. There's nothing to soak up excess liquid or counteract dehydration, and there are no vitamins. It's a sloppy scene in the stomach and a sloppy result in the toilet.

The solution is not only easy but delicious: eat more. I'd recommend my ingenious DOBE Policy (pronounced "doby"). DOBE (Drink On But Eat) is a hangover avoidance system. While you DO (Drink On) it's beneficial to pause briefly at times (eg, while opening new bottle) and supplement your liquid diet with water, green or herb tea. That's DOBE subclause (ii). Subclause (i) stipulates there are no rules, aside from the two critical parent clauses: DO (Drink On) and BE (But Eat).

There are many excellent foods to accompany drinking. For soaking up an excess of wine or spirits go for fibrous filling foods like bread, pasta, noodles, rice. Combine with vegies for vitamins, herbs spices garlic etc for flavour and health. Add cheese, meat, sausages or seafood for a real feast (and instant siesta).

Avoid dessert, unless you either simply can't resist

or haven't thrown caution to the wind for ages. For good health, not too much belly but way too much grog, nothing beats seafood with salad, accompanied by bread or pasta but preferably not cheese, and definitely not dessert. It's much easier for your stomach to tackle a few extra fish fillets or a tonne more salad and bread, than to embark on an entirely different project like dessert.

If you combine too many heavy-to-digest foods (cheese, meat, desserts, junk or fast foods) with drinking, you'll become very sluggish because your body is pre-occupied with digesting a concoction of challenges. Keep it simple and you'll have more energy. For an instant energy boost go for fruit or vegetable juice. Fresh salad is another pick-me-up and very effective hangover prevention or cure, as is fruit salad. Freshness and quality are important. See chapter XVII about growing your own.

Foods that require considerable time and effort to digest in the stomach are pretty smelly by the time they exit. If unrecognisable muck goes into your mouth, no wonder unpleasant shit eventually evacuates. When you eat chocolate, what is it? Handfuls of sugar? What does a sausage roll really consist of? What wondrous things make commercial breads stay squishy for ages? These things are not food. They're rubbish for the body to dispel.

Signs of poor diet or overloaded stomach include constipation or shit that's smelly, loose, sticky or heavy and black. Not good at all is green shit (suspect alcohol poisoning). Very good is honey-coloured shit that floats. Regularity means your digestive system is coping and a good diet normally results in a good shit every morning. Simple observation will tell you when you're getting it right with food and alcohol intake.

Most likely causes of constipation: too much food, no exercise, combination of many food types at once. Gentle digestive aids include wine, fruit, garlic, chilli, dried fruit, beans, wholegrain breads. Stomach antacids can be a quick fix. But if you really over-eat, it's going to take time to get through it. You can minimise this time by exercising (once you're able to move again) and by eating mainly fruit and vegetables (once you're able to eat again).

Foods that stick like superglue to plates when you do the dishes (melted cheese, meat fat, oily stuff) tend to stick with equal vigour to your insides. It's hard for stomach enzymes to churn them up. Things that slide off the plate or rinse off in cold water, like bread crumbs, fruit and salad, are cleansing in your body. It's easy for the enzymes to break them down. Animal products like steak and eggs take a long time to digest. When you consider they were dead long before you ate them, no wonder they're on the nose after spending a day or two inside your body. At least vegetarians aren't cemeteries.

If you want to eat a wide range of different foods in one day, give each meal time to digest. Half an hour to an hour is quite a bit of working time for the stomach, so a break between courses is very helpful (a little patience, big reward). A minimum of two to three hours is best between large meals, if you intend to fit into your clothes. Your stomach is best equipped for weighty foods when empty: cheese, eggs, nuts, icecream and desserts, chocolate, meat. The reason so many people end up feeling sick on Christmas Day is due more to the huge variety of foods eaten than the quantity.

Lightish combinations, such as antipasto platters, are no worries if there's a respectable gap (drinks break) between entrée and main. Soup is easy to digest, so it's a perfect starter. Salad accompanying anything aids digestion and fills you with goodness. Wine is great with food, not to mention before and after it. Cheese or dessert on a full stomach has a similar effect to a traffic accident on a busy freeway.

I could carry on endlessly with detailed analyses of particular foods and their metamorphosis as they journey through the body, but I've talked enough shit already. You'll learn more through your own studies, since we all have different diets and metabolisms. In every respect, our personal shit is unique. Don't fear it; learn from it.

XV
holidays

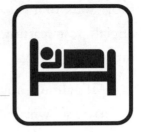

Drinking, eating, socialising, slothing — can be great, can be too much of a good thing; an indulgence overdose. We've all experienced the effects of too much food or alcohol, accompanied by too little exercise. It's easy to reach the point where mere anticipation of leaving the chair to fetch a tinnie is exhausting, and it can be stressful waiting for someone else to respond to your wails of, "Can you get me one while you're there?"

The longer the lazy phase continues, the harder it is to get motivated. Life can degenerate into a cycle of eating, sleeping and shitting that's not dissimilar to the habits of the earthworm. This could be an enormously positive thing for the future of life on earth, because if humans were as useful as earthworms the planet would be in fantastic condition.

I have a worm farm but don't want to be one. The eat/sleep/shit routine is perfect for worms but leaves humans flat and lifeless. What you need to do when you're on holidays and eating and drinking even more than usual, is keep up the exercise, even in reduced holiday-friendly form. An easy and convenient exercise is a

short walk of 15 to 20 minutes or more, especially beneficial post-feasting or as a metabolism boost in the
morning.

It's almost impossible not to put on weight during
holidays, so why not relax and let it happen. Keep up
enough exercise to feel alive and healthy and you'll enjoy
your holiday more. Keep emergency fat day clothes in
wardrobe, just in case (or your return to work may be
even more stressful, with buttons popping off and seams
ripping). Most importantly, learn how to spend more
time drinking without spending more time drunk.

Today I started drinking around midday. It's now
3.00 pm and I'm ready for my fourth tinnie. I'm not
drunk, because I've been drinking slowly. I'm not sober
either. An unhurried drinking pace has been easy
because I'm occupied. As well as writing this book, I've
had a fantastic experience with Edna, our semi-resident
echidna, just up the road. Australian animals are incredibly cute, and often exceptionally stupid. This absence of
wit can be due to lack of need (eg, echidnas only have
to find ants and, like many native animals, are predator-
free) or due to centuries of a fairly restricted vegetarian
diet often low in nutrients (think koalas).

Last year after about six weeks off for a fantastic
extended Christmas holiday, my mental capacity had
reduced to something not dissimilar to that of the koala.
And I loved it. My favourite pastimes, such as gardening

and cooking, require little mental arithmetic; more art and imagination really, and art doesn't have to be intelligent. So it's true, ignorance is bliss.

Right now I'm in the middle of another glorious long Christmas holiday, aiming for cerebral shutdown, expecting success. I'm so relaxed I wouldn't care if my brain fell out. This morning I harvested a few strawberries, handfuls of basil, parsley, rosemary, spring onions, a lettuce, stacks of spinach and a spectacular long beetroot in an S-shape.

Today's mental challenge is to make and eat excellent food, largely home-grown. I already have brilliant plans: avocado and salad sandwiches for lunch (after a few tinnies), root vegie soup and bread for dinner. I love cooking soup and other one-pot wonders, creating great flavours and making it up as I go. As mentioned in chapter XII (point ❷), the trick is to get the yumminess into the base: slowly simmered onions, carrots, silverbeet or swiss chards, flavoured with any combination of things like wine (last night's leftovers), anchovies, tamari, honey, herbs, chilli, garlic, spices, maybe adding salt, pepper, olive oil to taste near serving time. Like anything that is both creative and useful, cooking is very rewarding. A few wines, music, kitchen fun and cooking, plenty of eating and sleeping. Perfect.

Our fellow alcoholics, the pixies, like to come out after we're in bed and have their own food festivities;

exceptionally messy affairs which result in great splatterings of food and wine all over the kitchen and eating zones. I know this because I have to clean up after them next morning.

The temptation to drink oneself into oblivion is even greater on holidays than other times. If you clean your teeth before bed, remember some of the things you did after tea or make a feeble effort to tidy up after eating, you're pretty well on top of it. If you wake up not in a bed, fully dressed or with a throbbing headache, your holiday drinking patterns should be reviewed.

The key is time. Holidays are the perfect opportunity to slow down — physically, mentally. Slow your drinking pace down and you can enjoy the relaxing and happy effects of alcohol for even longer each day. Time is as precious as ever on holidays, because they don't last forever — a fact I'm so conscious of that even with weeks of holiday remaining, I'm panicking at the inevitable loss of freedom that must eventually greet me when I return to work, feeling as friendly as a newly-caged wild wallaby.

My outward attempts at a cool demeanour will no doubt give way to alarming outbursts of aggression if I become embroiled in verbal communications, so I might gaffer-tape my mouth for the first week back at work. Surrounding my workstation with gigantic trees and warning signs Enter at Your Own Peril could be another very practical way to ease myself back into the old routine, whilst also minimising harm to workmates.

Moments of exaggerated fear and panic, triggering the fight or flight response, are frequent: initial return to the big smoke; first pre-work night, often so intolerable as to cause last-minute holiday panic and drinking frenzy; wake up screaming because assume surrounded by fire, which turns out to be unfamiliar sound of alarm going off (contemplate ringing office to say flat on fire and therefore can't go to work, probably ever); the insult of getting out of bed before feeling ready; dressing up in ridiculous city outfits, more comical because all clothes have shrunk dramatically while not in use; overwhelmed by claustrophobia while commuting, only to be suffocated by greetings of workmates (none of whom are crying, so presumably they're on Prozac). Spend morning agonising over whether to go to doctor at lunchtime for my own Prozac, or vanish without trace.

I suspect my Mondayitis is aggravated by lack of alcohol. A popular concept here at my bush paradise (noticeably absent in my city workplace) is the "think I'll have one before lunch" routine. This urge emerges around midday, and is commonly followed by a procession of similar urges, culminating in a sort of collision between lunch and dinner. The desire for sobriety is no match for the deliciously pleasant effect of that first tinnie. The second is irresistible.

There's some hope of lunch before late afternoon if the urge is at least temporarily quashed after the second drink. Taking up the third urge option means you've probably traded willpower for frivolity, so enjoy that tipsy feeling and leave eating until ravenous. Don't stop drinking! Nothing is worse than a hangover while conscious. Remember the DOBE Policy.

Yesterday I did such a brilliant job of drinking at a sensible pace that lunch was at 4.00 pm and dinner at 11.00 pm, with such curtailed brain cell culling that I remember both! The downside is I'd feel more energetic today if I'd gone to bed earlier and slept longer. But I did enjoy a bottle of white and a bottle of red, without getting messy. No-one can dispute this because I was on my own.

Normally the drinking is faster, dinner and bed earlier, resulting in less overall alcohol consumption, more sleep, more energy and better health next day. But I don't feel sick because I feasted on good food. I don't have a headache because I don't smoke. I'm just going to be lazy. That's not a problem on holidays.

XVI
the private party

Mr X planted the private party seed in my mind, for which I thank him heartily. Most humans think parties have to involve more than one person. But to have your own super-exclusive private party is such a liberating and rich experience that no lifestyle is complete without it.

Unless you're having a garden party and communicating with plants, you'll find yourself talking much less at solitary parties, thus enhancing music enjoyment (and leaving mouth free for other things). You have total freedom regarding music selection and volume, for a delightful change. If you play an instrument you can make your own music, enjoying it whether fit for a king or worthy of earplugs.

There are absolutely no dress codes or customs, but wearing things you wouldn't normally wear to parties adds to the fun: eg, sexy underwear or nothing at all, maybe just shoes, a belt or some jewellery, a shirt or something extra-comfortable and daggy, possibly pyjamas, something old or stained that wouldn't fetch 10 cents in a garage sale. Be guided fully by the mood you're in, and change whenever you feel inclined.

There are in fact no rules at all. You can be happy and joyful or sad and crying. No matter what you do, no-one will be offended. You can dance or you can sit, you can cook or eat. You can wander around the house or the garden. You can even masturbate (although this could offend the neighbours, if you're indiscreet). You won't be arrested or get into a fight (unless defending yourself from neighbour invasion).

Just make sure you're very well stocked, so you can't possibly run out of your favourite types of alcohol and food. The last thing you'll want to do is go out (there's your appearance, for a start) and, being so unrestricted, private parties tend to outlast all expectations.

Dialling food is an alternative, but make sure you plan ahead, remembering that you need money and most delivery places close hours before you get hungry, plus you may need to talk without slurring incoherently, giggling or forgetting your order. It's also important to stay awake for the eternity it takes for the dubious feast to arrive.

Often private parties begin spontaneously, so planning ahead is replaced by an emergency dash to the bottle shop or deli. I cannot overstress the importance of stocking up as though hosting a nuclear fallout shelter. There's a carefree abandon about private parties that leaves one uninhibited, leading on occasion to frivolity and excess, even recklessness. Best to start early if you're having one on a week night.

If the phone rings or there's a knock at the door, you don't have to answer it (unless it's the delivery person) but you may if you wish. You can fart, hiccup, knock things over, smash glasses or plates (unintentionally, or for the undeniable thrill). You can look beautiful or a mess. You can behave perfectly or clumsily. You can dance like a ballerina, a rock star or a lunatic. You can stagger around and call it dancing. You can dance in darkness or candle light. Unnecessary objects (like furniture) can be moved to the edges of the room to create a spacious dance floor or general play area, doubling as padding if you find yourself hurtling unexpectedly towards the wall.

Sometimes I'm overwhelmed by affection for the people I love, and turn to the telephone. This can be a great idea, especially if the recipient of my jovial call is also drinking and unoccupied at the time, or it can be an embarrassing disaster. If only snippets of conversation are recalled next day, it's little comfort, and even more disconcerting if unsure who you were snippetting with.

Therefore, before you make the phone call, give a moment's thought to your state of sobriety and consider worst case scenarios. For example, your mother-in-law may not be receptive to your sudden generous warmth at midnight. Now may not be the time to propose to that interesting woman you met recently, whether your proposal is of marriage or just a — well, something less permanent. So think before you dial. If you can't find the number or have trouble operating the phone, this could be a sign that it's not the best thing to do right now.

The only other word of caution is to remember Safety First (see chapter XIII point ❺ on Time). If you absent-mindedly leave the gas on after a feast of home made pizzas, chop off a finger whilst making them or trip over the furniture in a moment of disorientation, there's no-one around to help. Of course, if no injuries result, you may welcome the lack of witnesses. Happily, we have an invaluable instinct to take extra care when alone, and there have been no accidents at my private parties (glasses, crockery, furniture and carpet excepted).

When the chips are down, a private party can be the best medicine. Many years ago I did an away job with some fellow court reporters in country New South Wales. I hadn't seen Mark for two weeks and he had booked our favourite restaurant for the night of my return. Come departure day, I was delirious with excitement.

Then disaster struck. My workmates and I headed for the country airport after a few post-work beers, but tragically our destination was so inconspicuous that we drove straight past it. As time passed and this realisation struck home, causing us to turn around and head back to find the airport at terrifying illegal speeds, my heart began to break. There was no way I could get back home that night.

The others had a different flight to catch, so they dropped me at a motel. I was bawling unashamedly by this stage. My senses were still intact sufficiently to quickly purchase half a dozen ales, in which to drown my sorrows. Better still, I had a Walkman and my Les Miserables album.

That night, after much crying and commiserating with Mark on the phone, I attached the music to my belt and sang along to Les Mis, time and time again, transported by the emotion and beauty of it all, while my own overemotional state dissipated. Dancing on the bed, with nothing on but belt, Walkman and headphones, I had a great party. I'm not sure why I danced mainly on the bed that night; things just happen at private parties, and everything that happens is okay. I woke up very happy.

After a few private parties you may find the common party uncomfortably overcrowded. They can also be noisy, smoky, with bad music, dubious company. There's often showing off and displays of superficiality, exaggerated or feigned affection, even outright aggression. You're in clothes you don't feel like wearing, talking to people you don't want to talk to, eating and drinking things you don't like, all the time trying to pretend you're enjoying yourself.

Then there's the problem of getting home, or worse still, cleaning up your own place. Private parties can be easily as messy as conventional ones, but at least the mess is yours. Best of all, there's no pretence at solo parties.

Common parties are the only time I'm in serious danger of drinking far too much and feeling ratshit next day. It's because if I'm not in the mood for it or don't want to be there, I drink fast in an effort to get happy, or out of nervousness or boredom. Plus these planned parties can be an imposition on valuable leisure time, having none of the flexibility of time and place that accompanies the private party.

I can metamorphose into an overexcited child at populated parties, leading to an excess of alcohol and affection. I'm also vulnerable to injuries, due to going-out shoes, foreign environments, faulty glasses, and the impossibility of staying awake in taxis — thankfully, because I'm usually petrified in them when sober. Sleeping in a taxi is not always a danger in itself, but controlling the body after such a slumber may be more than a shut-down brain can manage.

While common parties can be dangerous, they can also be great and memorable occasions. There's a time and place for all kinds of parties. Most people do themselves a disservice by attending only the standard type of party. If you're one of them, you've got so much to look forward to! And you can do it any time that suits you.

The private party devotee never fears being alone. Any time is a good time for a private party. Get to know yourself, dance with and date yourself, give yourself a dinner party, have a private garden party — whatever suits your mood. You'll be spontaneously laughing with and at yourself, not taking life too seriously, at your own exclusive parties. Treat yourself to a fresh perspective.

XVII
the vegie patch

The joy of growing your own vegies is understood by everyone who's given it a go. Eating is only one aspect. Watching cute little baby things evolve into sensational edible produce is reward in itself. As you water, prune, talk to and look after your little patch babies, you make a connection with them. You're reminded of the earth and the wonder of life on it. The plants and the worms, insects and birds they attract are all so alive, busy surviving and seeking to thrive. First you nourish them and then they nourish you.

And fresh vegies from your own organic garden will nourish you like nothing you can purchase. Their freshness ensures top quality taste and texture, maximum vitamins and minerals. It's because they're so nutritious that they taste so exceptionally good.

During the first half of the year, when our southern Victorian climate is most conducive to fruit and vegetable maturation, my body is invigorated by the extra goodness of an abundance of home-grown food. Most seasons we have an excess of apples, to the delight of workmates who marvel at their extra yumminess. This

sharing, admittedly, is due more to oversupply than gen-
erosity. Parting with heavenly home-grown produce can
bring out the Gollum in anyone.

Cooking interested me not, until Mark and I started our first vegie patch. Faced with beautiful produce
we had grown ourselves — initially potatoes and peas,
which seemed fascinating back then — I felt a responsibility to use them well. Terrified of ruining my vegies by
not preparing them in a yummy fashion, and acutely
aware that nothing is worse than boring vegetables, there
was only one thing for it: get cooking!

Soon I was beaming with confidence about the
deliciousness of our home-grown goods, so much so
that my grandparents were subjected to an awesome
pea feast on their memorable visit. For feeding me like
royalty through childhood, my gorgeous grandmother
was awarded a tower of peas! Imagine driving across
the Nullarbor for a pea party. They were too kind to
express any disappointment, and wisely devoted their
attention to the champers. The vision of pea mountains
on plates is still with me, and I'm hoping it's only
memory loss that those lonely pea mountains are unac-
companied.

Not only do I no longer astonish our occasional
visitors with truckloads of peas; I've evolved into an
enthusiastic gourmet chef. Mark and I feast like kings
here in the Otway Ranges. Planting, nurturing, harvest-

ing, cooking and eating occupies much of our country time. Perfect.

The most important thing to know about growing vegetables is it's really easy. The next thing is you don't need heaps of space. Vegetables, like humans, need food, water and sunlight. They do best with a nice balance of these factors, just like you do.

If you've never grown anything before, start with simple things. Lettuce, beetroot, potatoes, peas and beans, spinach and chards, leeks, spring onions — these are easy to grow, hardy, perfect green thumb cultivars. Every season you will learn more about growing things, not to mention the climate and environment you live in.

Best choices if your space is extremely limited: lettuce, chards, parsley, herbs. All can be grown in pots. Some herbs are so vigorous that pots are ideal: eg, mint, oregano, coriander. Check regularly to ensure they don't dry out. Buy a moisture metre. Herbs can look dry, even dead, only to spring back to life the moment they get a drink. You may have friends like this. If they're not the BYO type, they can be expensive because you have to supply them with alcohol instead of water. Watch out for the ones who "forget" their wallets.

Most of us real drinkers quickly ascertain which households are likely to "dry up" and we arrive with a sensible amount of grog; ie, more than could conceivably be consumed by the anticipated gathering. It's amazing how well the "I don't drink much" fraternity can adjust to new conditions and help with consumption, often to the point of bravely mimicking self-confessed heavy drinkers without any outward sign of reluctance.

The monetary downside of supplying the grog is more than compensated for by the mental upside, as fear of abruptly running out of alcohol can turn hair grey quicker than bankruptcy. At least bankruptcy takes an eternity and seems to rarely impact on lifestyle. By contrast, the threat of being unceremoniously and without warning thrust into a teetotalling session, with those who drank what you bought, is nearly as unnerving as the unwelcome shock of it actually happening.

I'd rather be drinking in the garden anyway. Mark and I never run out of alcohol, thanks to belonging to really good wine clubs and sensibly organising continual deliveries of wonderful wines. What a magnificent wine-making nation we are, and to think we produce drinkers of equal magnificence! As you can imagine, the wine clubs save us a fortune. It doesn't matter what type of grog it is: best to buy in bulk and save save save. For example, slabs of beer are a great bargain. After all, there are so many ways to spend money and so few that bring such pleasure.

When we first started joining wine clubs and ordering tasting packs and regular dozens, there lurked in our minds the fear of a sudden quite alarming and financially devastating increase in consumption. This was unfounded, we soon discovered. Easy availability of alcohol is not a danger; it's a blessing. An esky full of coldies, maybe some bourbon and cokes, ciders, plenty of red and white wines — this is standard for us, city or country (which means a lot of esky work in the bush).

Having a good supply of alcohol at all times has not resulted in a consumption blowout; rather, peace of mind. Before our sensible wine purchase planning, for example, if we bought a couple of bottles for the night we'd always finish them. Now that there's always wine available so that supply exceeds demand, we've settled into our natural drinking patterns without being influenced by externalities like the fear of running out (likely to cause panic and skolling) and the jealous obsession with ensuring that nobody else gets too much. Worse still, you may fall victim to temptation and greedily sneak a bit extra for yourself. This can lead to unwelcome feelings of guilt, plus you run the risk of getting caught red-handed and probably red-faced. It's all just tension that need not be endured.

I envy every cellar owner. Fortunately for all who know her, my mother has an excellent and well-stocked cellar. If you're not only too poor for a cellar but can barely afford bottled wine, there's some good quality cask wine around and you can enjoy the affordability of buying in bulk. My only concern with cask wine is the difficulty of assessing how much I've had. Relying on one's own optimistic consumption estimates can obscure a potentially hazardous and surprisingly rapid rate of cask depletion.

While gardening, keep your cask or bottle of wine or spirits indoors and there's a chance of not refilling every glass within seconds of emptying. It also means you have to move around a bit, and it's always good to stimulate the metabolism. As you know, due to all that good concentration on the serious stuff earlier, the alcohol needs to be processed and the body works harder when you're active. Remaining sedentary for long periods leads to physical and mental inertia.

The radio makes a perfect drinking companion in the garden: never complains, needs only positioning and occasional batteries, plus it's easier to change channels than get away from a common party bore. There are so many interesting and educational programs on the radio, and such a variety of views presented, including "radical" angles rarely explored on television. Hence gardening has become one of the most educational pursuits in my life.

Then there's sport and gardening. For the sports-loving alcoholic gardener, nothing beats an arvo outdoors with the footy on, or cricket etc. It's a healthier pursuit than staring at the box, and the commentary on radio is far superior.

It's also wonderful to listen only to the sounds of

the garden, in a relaxed and peaceful frame of mind. If you're searching for such a mood, classical music and gardens are beautiful companions. Even if your garden consists of a few pots on a window sill, it's still a living and growing garden and it's yours. When you add something home-grown to any dish, even a handful of herbs, you're contributing goodness and flavour.

Anyone with a front or back yard can grow a variety of vegies. They need good soil, not potting mix but real soil plus compost or manure, and water and sunlight. They will thrive if you love them. I was amazed when a friend of mine grew beautiful tomatoes and capsicums in near complete shade. She did it with TLC.

For many years Mark and I have been planting shrubs and grasses, vegies and fruit trees, plus a variety of gums and other natives. Baby trees need fencing, for wallaby protection, and as they grow so must the fences, until the trees are old and tough enough to go it alone. Whenever we replace old outgrown fences with new improved ones, the plant responds with a burst of growth. They adore the attention. And of course they like to be talked to and they love music.

Many vegies need staking for support, like tomatoes, capsicums, chillis and eggplants. Be careful not to damage roots by ramming in stakes close to their trunks. Ideally, put stakes in early; and next to, rather than into, the baby roots.

The difference between a thriving vegie patch and a poor one is usually the soil. "You are what you eat" applies to plants too. That's why hydroponically grown produce can look great but taste bland. All vegies thrive on well composted anything, especially animal manure. Straw makes fantastic mulch. It also attracts snails and slugs, infuriatingly, but there are various ways of dealing with these. There are even environmentally friendly baits on the market these days, bringing relief and happiness to people like me. It beats the hell out of dragging yourself from bed at night to find, catch and squash numerous horrible patch-munching slugs.

There are endless books on how to grow vegies. Growing from seed is very satisfying and opens up a wondrous world. Amongst the yummiest varieties I've grown are big sweet orange beetroots and exquisite Sunrise Hybrid cherry tomatoes, also orange. You won't find these in shops. Packets of mixed seeds are available — eg, lettuce, beetroot, chards, chillis. There's an exciting mystery factor when growing these, intensified by getting all the pots mixed up and losing track of what's where. Now I'm learning to differentiate the baby seedlings at an early stage, and can easily pick a weed from a newborn vegetable.

For the uninitiated, it's advisable to start with seedlings. Try seeds when you've built up some confidence. You can't go wrong with healthy seedlings unless you let them die of thirst or heat at a young age, or plunge them into a nutrient-free zone. If you purchase or make a compost bin (better still, two) you can have not only rich soil for vegies but make a positive contribution to the environment by turning your waste into something of great value, rather than contributing to landfill.

There's hardly any need for garbage once you start composting, because so many things are suitable for compost: all food scraps and leftovers, fruit and vegetable skins, tissues and toilet paper rolls, teabags, plus endless things from the garden like leaf material, dead plants, lawn clippings, supplemented by straw and animal manure. Even your own piss is good for compost (meaning urine of course; it would be a waste of alcohol).

Fantastic vegies can be grown with a minimum of time and fuss. If your soil is poor, try making a pile of straw and dynamic lifter (chicken shit) or sheep manure, layered together, then throw in some seed potatoes or whatever seedling you like, maybe planting into little holes filled with soil. You only have to watch and water after that. It's so easy. Liquid fertilisers are another way of supplementing poor soil, but they don't improve structure the way that composting does. Buying a bag of dynamic lifter and spreading it on top of the soil is a good way to launch a soil improvement program.

My enthusiasm on this topic borders on obsession, so it may be best to move on. Even if books or magazines about gardening bore you senseless, I'd urge you to try growing vegies — even just lettuce. The goodness in home-grown lettuce is amazing. It's an easy, fun way to eat healthy food. And the more alcohol you drink, the more important it is that you supplement your liquid diet with nutrient-rich foods (as all you good students fully appreciate by now).

XVIII
the half full glass

Isn't it challenging being patient with whingers? Most amazing is that so few perpetual grumblers have anything concrete to complain about. They may not be physically or mentally handicapped, their health may be fine and they may not be bankrupt, homeless, unloved or unappreciated, certainly not refugees or suffering from lack of freedom, opportunities or food, yet they're always whinging about something. Thus the half full glass can only be perceived as half empty.

Yesterday Mark and I were at a beautiful beach in a picturesque seaside port and aside from enjoying ourselves swimming, wining and dining, we planned to collect seaweed for our asparagus patch. Asparagus likes to have seaweed annually, although a good watering-in of salt is next-best if seaweed is impossible to obtain. As it turned out, our timing was bad, as there were people everywhere and we couldn't get a park near the beach. We were also concerned about the constabulary, because we have a suspicion that seaweed collection is illegal, but we're clinging to the ever-diminishing hope that it's not. Our desire not to break the law is second only to our desire not to get caught if we do. The seaweed expedition was cancelled at the last minute.

Well, you would think by my reaction that the whole town had run out of alcohol. I made myself miserable because I couldn't collect seaweed. How foolish. I'm on holiday in a perfect location, with my favourite person in the world, nothing at my disposal but time and enough money to have plenty of options. What an absurd tantrum to get upset over seaweed.

But people do it all the time. People get upset about nothing. It's as if we're searching for something to be angry or sad about, or for proof that we are uniquely badly done by in an uncaring world. Yet here in Australia most of us are in fact uniquely lucky. Not only are we not at war or starving and impoverished; we have an abundance of fresh food; a huge, spectacular country; a great variety of occupations to pursue. We have options.

You may not have a million dollars, you may work harder or longer than you wish. You may not be able to afford Dom Perignon. But if you're not sick and nor are your loved ones, if you're not in danger or a pauper, you could consider your life a privilege.

If hit by a bus tomorrow, I'd still be exceptionally lucky. I've already had an interesting and excellent life. So many people in this world have no opportunity for an education and little choice about how their lives evolve. Most people not only don't own a computer but will never experience a hot shower. Billions of people on this earth suffer from poverty, ill health and hunger.

My seaweed tantrum was shortlived. I soon realised I was being stupid, then chose to enjoy my day instead of ruining it. When younger, my emotional state was beyond control and it was hard to take an objective view. Now it's easy to bring a bit of perspective to bear. It's one of the advantages of experience and maturity, and there are very many others. You're less likely to notice them if you focus intensely on what you perceive as the negatives of ageing.

When you have a bit of a tantrum or maybe offend someone with an unkind remark or impatient attitude, it's easily remedied by getting over the tantrum or apologising where appropriate, then you can move on. The alternative is to wallow in negative emotions or work yourself into a frenzy of negative thoughts, thus turning a molehill into a mountain.

It's easy to get into bad mind habits. It might just be suffering from impatience when waiting for the train, for example, but why waste all that mental energy and upset yourself when you could be enjoying the opportunity to relax and let your mind wander, or read, file your nails, meditate — whatever you choose.

Of course it's easy being Mr or Ms Cool when getting our own way. I can be an absolute delight when I'm where I want, doing what I want. Children are the same. As adults, we learn how to disguise our feelings, but rarely how to control them. The big challenge is maintaining composure when what may be perceived as a crisis occurs: returning to work after holidays (very topical for myself right now, with one week to go); unable to go to favourite restaurant due to lack of funds; team loses Grand Final. Then there are real crises; emotionally destabilising experiences like heartbreak, family break-up, loss of loved one, terminal or debilitating illnesses.

It's appropriate to suffer difficult emotions when something sad or painful happens. Riding the storm and soldiering on to the best of your ability is the bravest option, but it's so easy to say and so hard to do. You may need help from others who have experienced similar misfortune, or from counsellors. There's no need to go through everything alone. Alternatively, you can wallow in self-pity; even dig a hole that you find yourself eternally stuck in.

It's normal to tally up a few battle scars, including deep emotional ones, during life. If you have the courage to respond to your personal challenges in as positive a way as the situation allows, well done. As fortunes change, you can wear every scar like a badge of honour and be proud of every year you have survived.

Whilst life may be punctuated here and there by misfortune, most of the time we have our routines, responsibilities and occupations, accompanied by the option to make the most of every day and every opportunity. You can grumble pitifully about all and sundry in the workplace, for example, and perceive only the empty part of every half full glass, but why torment yourself and your workmates unnecessarily? It's easy to see the negative side of things, but looking for the positive side is not only more uplifting, but way more rewarding and productive.

Negative thought patterns are largely just bad habits. It's easier for the brain to follow the same old routes, the path becoming more worn with each repetition. However, habits can be changed. It may take time and you may need help. I certainly did. When stressed out, I didn't realise I was worrying not only about every aspect of myself and my own life, but the rest of the world as well. It took ages to change some thought patterns, but it wasn't a difficult road once pointed in the right direction. I still monitor my thoughts, aiming to discard negative ones and focus on positive ones.

A big step on the road to improving your mental life involves stamping out the inner critic; that voice in your head that is hell bent on criticising you and then beating you when you're down. This frightening image or superego (so named because it's superimposed on your own natural and childlike ego) develops at a young age; a sort of hellish conglomerate of all the authority figures of youth.

The hardest part is identification. Once you've pinpointed the critic in your mind, you can embark on ignoring it, thus disempowering it and regaining control. The easiest way to differentiate the critic from the other players in your mind is the word "should". It's always dictating you should or shouldn't do things. If you listen to this voice and don't do what you should, off you go on a guilt trip. Feeling guilty makes you weak and vulnerable to further denigration by the power-crazed critic.

If you get into some heavy drinking and don't feel your best next day, the critic is ready to pounce. With a very "serves you right" air, a ghastly cycle of self-flagellation may begin, resulting in a day of misery, accompanied by unrealistic vows regarding future abstinence. When these vows are inevitably broken sooner or later, the critic has its chance to start the put-down routine again. The unrealistic vows are just future fodder for the critic.

Binge drinkers are often slaves to their inner critic, repeating the cycle of heavy drinking (naughty child cuts loose) then hangover with guilt trip (child admonished by critic) and plans for redemption (punishment by critic). But the ever-bubbly child can't be suppressed forever, so the pattern recurs. The more suppression the child has endured, the greater will be its next bid for freedom.

It's not ideal to be enslaved to your inner critic or inner child, but while the latter needs to be befriended so you can gain its trust and take the reins, the former needs to be silenced so you're free to grow unhindered by self-doubts. When you embark on a new project, there's usually a stage where something in your head tells you it's too hard or you're not capable. That's the inner critic. It doesn't want you to succeed because it's a parasite that feeds on your vulnerability. It only exists insofar as you allow it to dominate.

So how to kill it? As said, first identify it. This may take some time. Initially I didn't think I had an inner critic, because I was so accustomed to its presence in my head that I thought it was me. This is a common reaction, as we all like to think we're immune to common human frailties (eg, vanity, greed). Then when I did recognise it and became better at isolating it, the critic's trickiness and perseverance were daunting.

My therapist gave me weapons to wield against the critic, who is always older and bigger than you so you need special tactics. We used to stand with our hands against the wall and push against it with all our might, until we felt really strong and powerful. This feeling of strength is then harnessed, so it can be summoned when the critic launches an attack. We have to feel strong to resist it.

Because you're younger and less devious than the critic, it's no use trying to win an argument with it. You need to shut it up completely, by not listening. The best response is "shut up". Try also "fuck off". These are phrases that end a conversation rather than invite debate. That is what you're aiming to do; silence the critical talk and turn your mind to something positive or useful.

When you hear put-down comments in your head, suggesting you can't do things or you're hopeless or bad in whatever way, say "shut up" loudly in your head. Sometimes you need to work at it for a while. You've probably been letting the critic lecture you for years, and it's not easy to break old habits. With time, you'll get better and better. Keep telling it to shut up, shouting at it if necessary. Eventually your mind will be able to move on and absorb itself in your current activity.

All this heavy talk in a book about drinking. Why? Because a huge number of drinkers and alcoholics torment themselves with guilt trips and other modes of self-flagellation. There's no need. If you free your mind from these negative patterns, you can enjoy your activities more, not to mention your drinking.

XIX
lifestyle

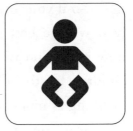

It's easy for me to be a healthy alcoholic because, by choice, I have no children. I'm lucky to have kids in my life (nephews and a niece) but I've never wanted the responsibility of my own offspring.

Not having children means not getting up early on weekends or during the night; not being exhausted; having more leisure time. I'm free to spend time gardening and cooking, so it's easy for me to prepare very healthy food. If you're a parent there are other people to consider and things more important to think about than when and what to drink. There are also more financial commitments.

Assuming parenthood means less money and less time, combined with a desire to present a reasonably sober image for the children, it's no wonder parents are inclined to reduce their alcohol intake. It's demanding being a parent. I have nothing but admiration for them, and heartily congratulate anyone who makes the commitment. The rewards are of course enormous. But like many worthwhile pursuits, discipline and effort are required.

So if your reality includes raising children, naturally it will be best for everyone if you're realistic about how much and when you can afford to drink. After the children go to bed is a good time. And if you're not drinking as much as you used to, or plan to do once the kids grow up, maybe you can treat yourself to really good quality stuff when you do. But if you can't afford the best you'll enjoy it anyway, bearing in mind the children are in bed. If you don't have much drinking time, you can drink more quickly and enjoy the uplifting effects in the time you do have.

It's natural for parents to embrace a disciplined lifestyle, and children respond well to routine. Balancing the discipline with letting your hair down can be an effective means of releasing tension. Alcohol is a great vehicle. Without doing anything illegal or spending too much money or time, you can lift your spirits and elevate your mood, laugh and enjoy yourself, forget about the daily grind.

Sharing a bottle of wine with a friend doesn't take long (not long enough, generally) but the memory might last forever. You're more likely to recall loved ones, friendship and great times on your death bed, than the innumerable occasions when you rocked up to work and then worked.

If you want to be a healthy drinker you have to keep your drinking in tune with your lifestyle. You want harmony rather than conflict. While drinking and gardening mix well, drinking and deep sea diving don't. As long as you're honest with yourself about how much you like to drink and realistic about how much is appropriate in the given circumstances, it's not hard to find a balance that complements your lifestyle.

If you create problems for yourself while drinking, like getting aggressive or behaving unreasonably, spending more than you can afford, ignoring your responsibilities, this self-destructive behaviour may be the result of unresolved problems or issues in your life. Suppressed problems will surface whenever given half a chance, and alcohol can be that opportunity. Giving up alcohol may fix the inappropriate behaviour but it won't fix the problem, which will continue to fester until attended to.

It's very tempting to blame every personal misfortune or inconvenience on someone or something else. Judging by the number of times my nephews plea "it's not my fault" and "it's not fair", this is instinctive. Trouble is, it doesn't get results. If you want something done or a situation changed, the best way to get action is to launch into it.

If you choose to take responsibility for yourself, rather than blame what happens in your life on external factors, you become empowered. You may not be able to change others or even change particular scenarios, but you can change yourself. You can change your perspective. You can be an alcoholic and deny it or give yourself a hard time about it; but equally you can be an alcoholic by choice and enjoy a drinking lifestyle.

I once said to my auntie, while enjoying a happy reunion over a few wines, "I'd do much more in my life if I didn't drink," to which she replied, "Yes, Cindy, but you wouldn't have so much fun." She drinks very moderately herself, but is clearly very perceptive.

Just because you're a drinker doesn't mean you can't be any number of other things as well, or even do constructive things and drink simultaneously. Be practical about which activities are drinking friendly and which aren't.

XX
dinner parties

Dangerous. First, pre-party panic, at worst including dieting, shopping and hours of preparation. The awkward arrival, guests dolled up and feigning a relaxed mood, desperate for a calming drink, especially those who didn't have any before leaving home (not that I've ever fallen for that, thanks again to a tip from Mr X).

After a couple of drinks things have dramatically improved, to the point where you're starting to enjoy yourself and everyone seems friendly and interesting. This pleasurable trend continues for the next few drinks, as you become more and more friendly and interesting yourself, or at least that's what you think.

Food shuts people up for short periods, both a relief and potential embarrassment, but it also has a relaxing effect on anyone who doesn't have an eating disorder, and provides essential vitamins etc. Enjoy the food bit. DOBE — Drink On But Eat — it's your only hope.

Hang around for long enough after the post-meal coffees and subsequent port or anything whatsoever that contains alcohol, and things are bound to get sleazy, slovenly or hilarious. Dancing is a great way to burn up the excess of calories you have hopefully consumed, plus keep the liver activated. You don't need me to tell you this, now that you're metabolism experts. Putting your drink down, to devote yourself exclusively to dancing, is very health-conscious, but you've got nil chance of finding it afterwards.

There comes a time when leaning on your dancing partner is not so much a display of affection as a physical necessity. Bodily contact is a pleasure sport as well as a survival tactic at dinner parties, because sooner or later the conversation becomes repetitive, difficult to follow or completely stupid, and the music is so loud that staying awake is unavoidable (unless you've really overdone it and lose consciousness; a state you'll be longing for next day).

A great time may be had by all, but dinner parties are costly, physically and financially. Those holding the dinner party spend a fortune on the latest groovy foods and quality grog, aiming to impress. Attendees splash out on new outfits and showy wines. All that expensive alcohol would normally prevent a hangover, but at a dinner party everyone drinks too quickly, due to excitement and stress. As for the poor smokers, they can barely draw oxygen through the tar next day.

If all guests make it home safely, danger still lurks. Before I even began to drink it was obvious that alcohol deserved respect. The aftermath of dinner parties was my first clue. Dinner party lovers tend to suffer big time. I suppose I did too, in my twenties, when pushing the limits was irresistible. But no longer. Probably because I don't hold or go to dinner parties.

If they're part of your life, take a few precautions. Be extra healthy the day before, FAP if possible (that's fuck-all-piss, introduced in chapter VI). I've rarely achieved this, probably due to rule aversion, but it's sensible if you can swing it. Take a couple of milk thistle tablets or other liver tonic before going out, with lots of water, and when you get home if you're still conscious, and again next morning.

You'll probably still be drunk when you wake up. Enjoy that bit, because unless you're up for hair of the dog, it won't last. Drink copious water and fruit juice, and/or eat fruit. Any fruit or vegetable juice is ideal. With any luck, by the time you're sober, you'll be less dehydrated. If you want a real detox, carrot and beetroot juice is sensational. It can be accompanied by something green like spinach or celery, and is delicious with ginger. It's serious though, so don't try your first detox when there's more alcohol than blood in your veins (unless you want to vomit).

Above all, keep your mind positive and don't dwell on how you feel. You'll be right, mate. Just look at you; a real Aussie.

XXI
cheers

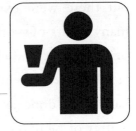

As the sun set in Marla, often in spectacular fashion in the red desert, most nights Deane, Mark and I would barely notice because we were too busy finishing the transcript. By about 7.00 pm Mark and I had a hard-earned thirst that we weren't prepared to deny any longer, so out came our favourite post-work drinks. Deane understood, and usually joined us. Although we had to work on into the night for one, two or too many more hours, we knew we needed to relax a bit and try to enjoy ourselves in a difficult situation, to maintain our sanity. Sensibly pacing ourselves, it was possible to drink and work for however long it took.

We were very pleased with the respect we earned in Marla. One barrister described it as a Rolls-Royce service, which of course we knew it was, but the compliment made us feel great. No-one complained that the transcript was delivered by a tinnie-drinking court reporter in jovial spirits. I think they liked it. So much better than a grim-faced angry person, desperate for a drink and without a sense of humour.

Normally I don't drink and work at the same time,

but these were extreme circumstances. There were so many hours of work that it was either work and drink, or just work. The choice was obvious. It wasn't difficult at all to drink while working, because we knew what had to be done and paced ourselves accordingly. It's a matter of being realistic.

Surviving Marla gave me that inspirational feeling of being able to do anything. Giving up smoking can have the same effect, like reaching any goal that's difficult to attain. My normal life is a perpetual holiday compared to our time at Marla. But what great desert memories we have.

Funny how the most difficult experiences can also be the best. If it's possible to rise magnificently to the occasion when called upon, it must be possible to achieve or do or experience more in ordinary life.

Drinking doesn't have to mean getting nothing done. It didn't stop us getting the job done in Marla. Don't think that because you're a drinker you can't simultaneously do and be countless other things. You can keep drinking but get healthy at the same time. Here's to health. Cheers!

Notes

Notes

Notes

Notes

Would You Like To Be Published?

Self publish through a successful Australian publisher.

Brolga provides:

- Editorial appraisal
- Cover design
- Typesetting
- Trade distribution

Enquiries to:

Brolga Publishing Pty Ltd
PO Box 12544, A'Beckett Street
Melbourne, 8006, Victoria, Australia

Fax: (03) 9671 4741
Email: bepublished@brolgapublishing.com.au
ABN: 46 063 962 443

Order your copy of:

Fit, Healthy & Intoxicated
Qty

ISBN 1-920785-33-7   RRP $24.95   .....

Postage & Handling $8.00   .....
within Australia

TOTAL★ $_____
★ All prices include GST

Name: _____

Address: _____

_____

_____

Phone: _____

Email Address: _____

Method of Payment:

❑ Money Order ❑ Cheque ❑ Bankcard ❑ MasterCard ❑ Visa

Cardholders Name: _____

Credit Card Number: _____

Signature:_____ Expiry Date: _____

Allow 21 days for delivery.

Payment to:

Better Bookshop

PO Box 12544 A'Beckett Street, Melbourne, 8006

Victoria, Australia

Fax: (03) 9671 4741

Email: betterbookshop@brolgapublishing.com.au

ABN 14 067 257 390